CHINESE
MASSAGE
THERAPY

Chinese Massage Therapy

A handbook of therapeutic massage

Compiled at the
Anhui Medical School Hospital/China

Translated by
Hor Ming Lee & Gregory Whincup

Introduction by
Ronald Puhky, M.D.

SHAMBHALA

BOULDER 1983

Published in the U.S.A. by
Shambhala Publications, Inc.
1920 13th Street
Boulder, Colorado 80302

Produced by
Cloudburst Press Ltd.
©1983 by Cloudburst Press Ltd.
All rights reserved.

Distributed by Random House.

Printed in the United States of America.

Library of Congress Cataloging in Publication Data

T'ui na liao fa. English.
Chinese massage therapy.

Translation of: T'ui na liao fa.
1. Massage. I. Lee, Hor Ming. II. Whincup,
Gregory. III. An-hui i hsüen yüan. Fu shu i yüan.
T'ui na liao fa pien hsieh hsiao tsu. IV. Title.
[DNLM: 1. Massage. WB 537 A596t]
RM723.C5T8413   1983   615.8'22   82-42677
ISBN 0-87773-225-6 (pbk.)
ISBN 0-394-71423-7 (Random House : pbk.)

CONTENTS

CHAPTER I

PRINCIPLES OF MASSAGE THERAPY
3

CHAPTER II

TECHNIQUES OF MASSAGE THERAPY
8

CHAPTER III

ACUPOINTS COMMONLY USED
IN MASSAGE THERAPY
60

CHAPTER IV

HOW TO USE MASSAGE THERAPY
72

APPENDIX

INDEX

CHAPTER V

CLINICAL APPLICATIONS OF MASSAGE THERAPY
84

CHINESE
MASSAGE
THERAPY

INTRODUCTION

It has been my privilege to have worked on this text, translated from the original Chinese. My task was to check the accuracy of the medical terminologies used, especially to render them into the more current medical usage from the somewhat archaic terms obtained in the process of direct translation. I did this without changing the concepts and attitudes towards treatment of the original Chinese authors. I also reviewed the terminologies used in the sections pertaining to acupressure and, particularly, made some of the descriptions of point locations a little easier to follow. However, in this area particularly, direct learning under supervision is the only really effective way to learn acupuncture point locations. This area of the text remains then, a guide to further study.

It is my feeling that the clinical work in massage therapy done in China is without equal in the world. The extremely effective work in this modality follows from the over three millenia of experience in traditional Chinese medicine in treating internal conditions of the body by manipulating, pressing, rubbing, heating, or needling surface areas of the body.

This text, then, supplies the Western reader with an introductory perspective on the methods of and indications for Chinese massage therapy.

The overall basis of the text is for the treatment of a variety of pathological conditions from minor to severe. As such its primary audience will be health care professionals: massage therapists, physiotherapists, naturopaths, chiropractors, nurses and physicians. Indeed, many of the conditions described require prior medical work-up and investigation while some require actual hospitalization; in this instance massage is just one of the many therapies utilized.

There is a still wider audience for this book, however. The general public has been over recent years demanding access to information in health areas formerly held exclusively by professionals. This includes information about effects of therapy, drugs, non-surgical alternatives, nutrition, methods of preventive medicine, and a whole host of related areas in health maintenance and general self-improvement.

Since massage applies itself very well as a general tool for relaxation and promotion of overall well-being, the interested and responsible layperson should find much useful information in this book about general methods of massage. Even the more clinically oriented sections will allow him or her to be aware of the therapeutic possibilities of the Chinese massage methods, inspiring the seeking out of practitioners who have a knowledge of such methods.

It is my hope that both my colleagues in Western medicine and the interested lay reader will find this book a useful contribution to their store of knowledge.

Ronald Puhky, MD; Bachelor of Acupuncture,
College of Traditional Medicine, U.K.; Diplomate, College
of Traditional Chinese Medicine, Peking.

Peking, People's Republic of China, April 8, 1982

CHAPTER I

PRINCIPLES OF MASSAGE THERAPY

Massage therapy has been gradually developed by the working people of China through a long process of working, living, and of struggling with disease. It is simple and easy to use and its particular effectiveness in treating certain common ailments has gained it wide acceptance among working people.

How does massage cure disease? It is generally considered that massage therapy has the ability to regulate nerve function, to strengthen the body's resistance to disease, to flush out the tissues and improve circulation of blood, and to make the joints more flexible.

1. *Regulating nerve function:*
The nervous system links all parts of the body, influencing the function of every part and every organ. Imbalanced nerve function, or increases in nerve excitement or nerve inhibition can all cause the malfunctioning of certain organs, resulting in disease. There is the pathogenic principle: "If *yin*[1] predominates over *yang*[2], then a *yang* disease appears; if *yang* predominates over *yin*, then a *yin* disease appears." The use of massage therapy techniques

---

1. *Yin:* the negative principle associated with contraction.
2. *Yang:* the positive principle associated with expansion.

has a reflexive effect on nerve functions, causing the excitatory and inhibitory processes of the nervous system to reach a relative equilibrium (i.e., bringing the *yin* and the *yang* into relative equilibrium). And this, in turn, produces a medical effect. For example: when a headache or toothache is present, massage applied on a corresponding acupoint[3] (such as the *hegu*[4] point) kills the pain immediately. This occurs because the massage creates a new stimulation point, easing or dispelling the sensation of pain in the original location. This phenomenon is called the "pain-shifting method." With hypertensive patients who exhibit such symptoms as dizziness and headache (said to be caused by too much *yang* in the liver), massage brings about a temporary drop in blood pressure. This is because the massage techniques cause the peripheral blood vessels to dilate through nervous reflex action. This type of regulative process is called "suppressing the liver's *yang*."

Also, for example, where there is a common cold or flu caught due to wind or cold, the pores of the skin are blocked, so that no perspiration can pass through them. Consequently, the body temperature rises and there is tiredness all over the body, as well as headache and discomfort. After massage is applied, the whole body reacts with perspiration, and the symptoms abruptly disappear. This phenomenon is called "relieving the surface of the body."

In the case of acute urine retention, applying massage on the lower abdomen and on a corresponding acupoint (such as the *qihai*[5] point) triggers bladder contraction, and the discharge of urine.

In recent years, there has been some experimental evidence to substantiate that massage therapy does produce such results as those mentioned above. For example, massage applied to the neck and upper back or lower back regions did increase the flow of blood to the internal organs associated with the corresponding section of ganglia. We have made some experimental investigation of the effects of massage on gastric activity. These showed that

---

3. Acupoint: one of a large number of specific points on the body at which massage or acupuncture are applied to produce specific system effects.
4. *Hegu:* an acupoint located on the back of the hand between the bones of the thumb and index finger. See Diagram 59, p. 65.
5. *Qihai:* an acupoint point just below the umbilicus. See Diagram 58, p. 63.

massage applied to the *weishu*,[6] *pishu*[7] and *zusanli*[8] acupoints did indeed increase the strength of gastric activity. Where gastric activity has already been functioning in a fortified state, and the same method of massage is used, it leads conversely to the inhibition of gastric activity. This demonstrates the regulatory use of massage, which produces different effects when applied with the stomach function in different states. We have applied the outcome of these experimental observations in our clinical practice and obtained further verification. When the above method was applied in a postoperative patient suffering from intestinal obstruction, the intestinal peristalsis returned to normal. Also, the use of this method has slowed intestinal peristalsis and dispelled the pain in a patient affected with enterospasm.

2. *Strengthening the body's resistance to disease:*

Massage therapy can improve general physical condition, and strengthen the body's resistance, resulting in the prevention and curing of disease. The underlying principle of treatment is "support the good and expel the bad." For example, in the case of a patient with rheumatoid spondylitis, not only does massage therapy make the stiffened vertebral column more flexible and lessen pain, but after a period of massage treatment, the patient's complexion turns from gray to rosy, and better appetite and weight gain occur. As general physical condition improves, the effect of treatment is further promoted. Also, in a patient with gastroptosis, massage therapy not only improves gastro-intestinal function, eliminating a series of symptoms in the gastro-intestinal tract, but it also raises the whole body's muscle tone to a higher level. Consequently, the general situation is improved, and the effect of the original treatment is augmented and consolidated. Again, in certain cases of infantile pneumonia, though there was a long course of treatment with antibiotics, a murmur in the pulmonary area persisted, and the whole body was weak. After massage therapy, the murmur soon died out, and gen-

---

6. *Weishu:* an acupoint on the back, beside the lower end of the spinal process of the 12th vertebra. See Diagram 59, p. 65.
7. *Pishu:* an acupoint on the back, beside the lower end of the spinal process of the 11th vertebra. See Diagram 59, p. 65.
8. *Zusanli:* an acupoint on the outer edge of the tibia, just below the knee. See Diagram 60, p. 69.

eral condition also gradually improved. This illustrates how massage therapy mobilizes the body's internal defenses against disease.

Based on the fact that after massage treatment the skin in the area appears reddened, we made experimental observations of skin temperature before and after massage. The findings showed that skin temperature rose both in the local area, where the massage had been applied, and in areas distant from the massaged spot. This implies that massage can accelerate metabolism, and cause dilation of peripheral blood vessels, increased blood circulation, and strengthened resistance against invasion by noxious influences. In addition, observations were made of the effects of massage on red blood-cell count, white blood-cell count, the ability of the white blood-cells to destroy bacteria, and the serum complement values. The results demonstrated that, after massage was applied, each of these indices was raised above its previous level. This shows how massage can help the body to protect itself against disease.

3. *Flushing out the tissues and increasing circulation of the blood, making the joints more flexible:*

The direct effects of massage therapy are most easily seen externally in the treatment of localized ailments. For example, for sprained limbs, bruises and local hematomatic pain, massage therapy can flush out the tissues and improve circulation of the blood, replacing spilled blood cells with new ones, completely removing the localized collection of the leaked blood and causing the swelling pain to fade. In clinical observation, we found that to reduce a swelling means, in effect, to stop pain. This accords with the principle: "Where the blood does not flow, there is pain; where the blood flows, there is no pain."

In all types of paralysis resulting from muscular atrophy, massage therapy can speed up the restoration of normal muscle tone, and strengthen the muscles. This is known as: "Clearing the energy-system and strengthening the flesh and bones." Also, in cases of joint stiffness due to any variety of causes, massage can directly increase the degree of activity in the stiffened joints. In the case of articular rigidity caused by rheumatoid spondylitis, our clinical observations show that the joint is not irreversibly stiff as mistakenly believed in the past. In fact, the joint is as if "rusted," and therefore some of the passive methods of manipulation used in massage will gradually loosen the rusted joints.

We have also studied a comparatively large number of cases of protruding lumbar intervertebral disk ("slipped" disk). We found that the mechanical force applied during massage returned the protruding area to its proper place. Based on these findings we have improved the methods used in this massage, and have further advanced the effectiveness of the treatment.

The above represents an introduction to the basic principles of treatment by massage therapy. Just as matter evolves, so does man's knowledge. Through actual practice our knowledge is continuously developed and increased, making massage therapy an even more effective method for the prevention and cure of disease.

Furthermore, it must be pointed out that the successful outcome of massage therapy will be greatly enhanced by a positive relationship between the practitioner and the patient. In massage therapy, it is necessary to have close coordination between them. This is especially true for certain ailments where the patient has to undertake a long-term program of self-massage and exercise to go along with professional treatment. These consolidate, and improve the therapeutic effect of the treatment. Therefore, in the course of treatment, it is important to bring the subjective motivation of both practitioner and patient fully into play, and to establish confidence in the treatment and healing processes.

CHAPTER II

TECHNIQUES OF MASSAGE THERAPY

Section I: Commonly Used Techniques

In Chinese medical literature there is abundant information about massage techniques. Massage-therapists from all parts of China have combined their clinical experience, and in the primary or secondary aspects of these techniques, each one has his own particular way of doing things. Below is an introduction to our commonly-used techniques.

1. Press Method

The press method is a form of massage which uses the palm or the fingers to press on a certain part of the body. There are various ways to apply the press, such as with one hand, both hands, elbow, etc. When the press method is used one must gradually go from light to heavy, so that the patient feels a definite pressure, but no pain. At the close of the press method it is not desirable to release the pressure too suddenly. Instead, the pressure should be gently reduced. The press method may be applied continuously for a comparatively long space of time, or intermittently, at a fixed rate. After the press method has been applied, some other techniques must be added in combination with it. The effects of the press method can be felt as shallowly as just on the surface of the skin, or as deeply as in the bones and internal organs. The amount of pressure used can be adjusted as necessary.

The press method is divided into three different forms: palm press, finger press, and elbow press:

a) *Palm Press Method:* The palm press method involves using the palm to apply pressure to an affected area of the body. Included are the single-palm press, two-palm press, and two-palm opposed press. The palm press is generally applied where there is an extensive area of pain, as in lumbago, or abdominal pain. (See Diagram 1.) If the entire head is in pain then the two-palm opposed press (see Diagram 2) is used. In pressing on the abdomen, the pressing hand must follow the rise and fall of the patient's respiration. Doing so will prevent the patient from feeling discomfort. Sometimes the practitioner first rubs his palms until they become very hot, and then presses on the painful area. This has been found effective.

DIAGRAM I

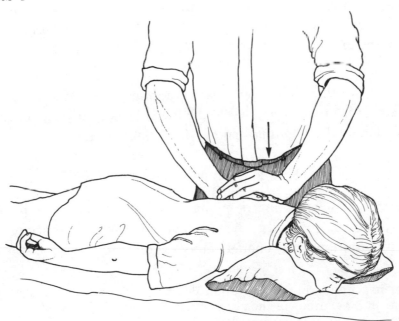

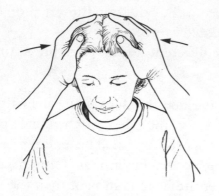

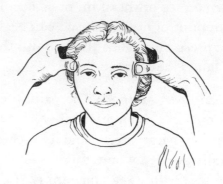

DIAGRAM 2   DIAGRAM 3

b) Thumb Press Method: When applying the thumb press method, press the flat of the thumb on a meridional acupoint (an acupoint situated on a meridian of the body's energy system) or on the site of the pain. While pressing, a suitable force must be applied, trying to avoid as much pain as possible. In the thumb-press method the single-thumb press and the two-thumb opposed press may be used. For an ache in the the forehead, for example, the two-thumb opposed press is applied to the *taiyang*[1] acupoints in the temples. (See Diagram 3.)

c) Elbow Press Method: The elbow press is applied either at an acupoint or at a site of pain. It is properly applied to the lower back, buttocks, or to certain acupoints such as the *huantiao*[2] point. (See Diagram 4.)

2. Rub Method

The rub method uses the fingers or the palm. There are single-handed and also two-handed rub methods. They involve rubbing the surface of the skin with a circular motion. Only enough force is applied to affect the skin and the

---

1. *Taiyang:* an acupoint in the depression about a finger's width outside a point between the outer canthus of the eye and the tip of the eyebrow.
2. *Huantiao:* an acupoint on the buttock, between the highest point of the trochanter and the sacral hiatus. See Diagram 59, p. 65.

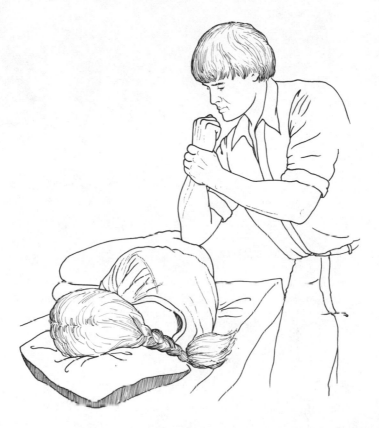

DIAGRAM 4

subcutaneous tissues. The force of the rub should go from light to heavy, and the rate of the rub movement depends on what the condition of a disease requires; it should be somewhere between 30–40 and 200 times a minute.

The rub method is often used at the beginning of a massage, or performed just after the press method. Rub techniques generally include thumb, palm and palm-heel rub methods.

a) Thumb Rub Method: This refers to rubbing with the flat of the thumb on a certain area of the body, or on an acupoint. It can be done with one thumb or with both thumbs at the same time. When using both thumbs, attention must be paid to coordinating their action, and their pressure must be identical. Be sure that the thumbs meet the skin squarely. Have the other four fingers slightly spread apart, with knuckles slightly bent so that during the rubbing the fingers do not touch the skin. Rub with a circular motion, mov-

DIAGRAM 5

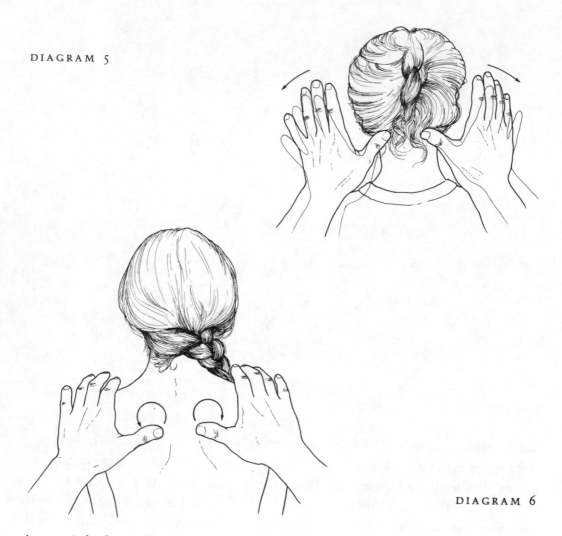

DIAGRAM 6

ing mainly from the wrist. Generally, this method is used for headache, or poor eyesight, rubbing on the head and face, the back of the neck, and on the *fengchi*[3] acupoints at either side of the base of the skull. (See Diagram 5.) On the back and the abdomen, the two-thumb circular rub can also be used. (See diagram 6.)

---

3. *Feng chi* acupoints: the depressions located at the base of the skull between the mastoid bone and the trapezius on each side. See Diagram 59, p. 65.

b) *Palm Rub Method:* The palm rub method is carried out with the palm of the hand lying flat on the body. Generally only one hand is used. Rub slowly in a clockwise direction, maintaining even pressure.(Diagram 7.) The palm rub is generally suited for larger areas of the body, and is used mostly on the chest, the abdomen, and the back. When indigestion occurs in children and the chest and ribs are bulging, the second rib section is rubbed. When a child has pain from over-eating, the abdominal area can be rubbed. For lumbar strain, the lower back region can be rubbed.

DIAGRAM 7

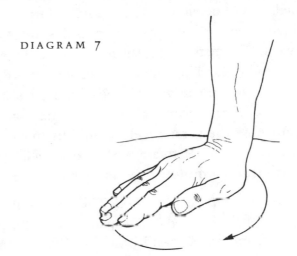

c) *Palm-Heel Rub Method:* Rub with some force, using the muscular pads on either side of the base of the palm. Keep the fingers and the thumb raised upward off the skin surface, with all the finger joints slightly bent. Swing left and right from the wrist. (Diagram 8.) Both hands can be used alternately. Push forward at the same time as you swing from left to right at a rate as fast as 100 to 200 times a minute. The palm-heel rub is good for the lower back region, as in cases of backache or flu. When these are present, the lower back region is massaged up and down. This technique produces a sensation of warmth, making the patient feel comfortable and relaxed.

DIAGRAM 8

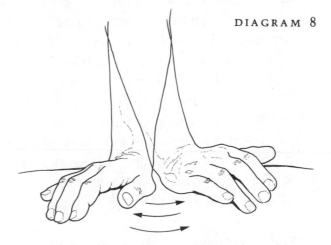

3. Push Method

In the push method either the fingers and thumb or the palm is used to push back and forth or left and right on the skin. The depth that the massage reaches will depend on the degree of force used. It can be as shallow as the subcutaneous tissues and the muscles, or as deep as the bones and internal organs. During massage, the force applied should be gradually increased from light to heavy. The amount of force used is determined by the nature of the ailment and the individual characteristics of the patient. Especially with those who are receiving their first massage treatment, frequent inquiries about how the person feels should be made, as well as observations of his reactions, in order to allow the proper adjustments. Frequency is generally 50–150 times a minute, beginning slowly, and gradually increasing speed.

a) Flat-Thumb Push Method: The flat-thumb push method is also called the "spiral push method." The pad of the thumb is used to stroke the skin surface, moving forward in a single direction. While pushing forward, the thumb has to exert pressure. But when moving back, the knuckles of the thumb must be slightly flexed and the back of the thumb carried back along the skin to the starting place. On the forward push, the knuckles of the other fingers should be slightly bent. On the return, extend them straight. Do not apply any force with the fingers, but use them only to help maintain position. (See Diagram 9.) Repeat over and over again, increasing speed.

Skill in this technique must be developed with long practice, so that the fingers and the thumb become strong enough, and the joints of the fingers, the thumb, and the wrist become very flexible. Then the force of massage can be varied exactly as desired. The flat-thumb push can be done with one hand or with both hands alternately or simultaneously. When both thumbs are used simultaneously, they go to the left and to the right from a meridional acupoint. This technique is also called the "divergent push method."

The flat-thumb push method has wide application. It can be applied to the head, the back, or the limbs. In general, it is most often used in the head and back areas, as shown in Diagram 10. Where pain is present in the forehead, the divergent push method can be applied at the *yintang*[4] and *zuanzhu*[5] acu-

---

4. *Yintang* acupoint: a point situated between the eyebrows. See Diagram 58, p. 63.

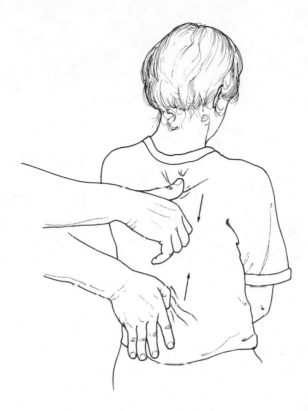

DIAGRAM 9

points of the brow ridge. The divergent push method is also applied on the shoulder and at the *dazhui*[6] acupoint. There is another type of divergent-push method called the "muscle-dividing" method. This utilizes a force deep enough to reach the muscular layer. In this case the divergent push follows the direction of the musculature. This pushing technique has been found most effective in sprains of the back and the loin.

b) *The Side-of-the-thumb Push Method* is also termed the *"shaoshang*[7] push method."* This technique resembles the flat-thumb push. The only difference between them is that when pushing out, the force is applied with the

---

5. *Zuanzhu* acupoint: a point located at the medial end of the eyebrow. See Diagram 59, p. 65.
6. *Dazhui* acupoint: a point between the spinous process of the 7th cervical vertebra and that of the 1st thoracic vertebra. See Diagram 59, p. 65.
7. *Shaoshang:* an acupoint on the outer side of the thumb, at the lower corner of the nail.

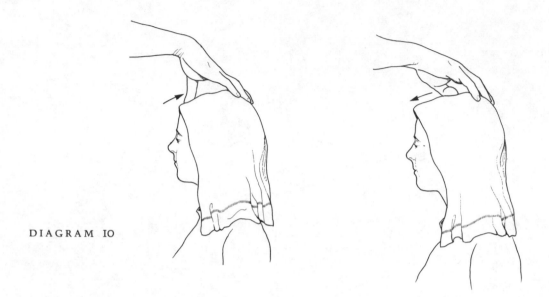

DIAGRAM 10

lateral surface of the thumb (i.e. the *shaoshang* acupoint). This method of massage is often used on the *pitu*[8] line in the thumb and the *sanguan*[9] line of the forearm, and also on the head and limbs (when the extremities are in a state of paralysis).

c) The Thumb-tip Push Method: This kind of manipulation is usually employed on an acupoint, or on the main site of pain in an illness. During the pushing, the tip of one thumb is used. It moves such a small amount, that it appears to have been attached to the acupoint. The wrist is bent and hangs downward. The joints of the thumb bend and extend quickly. Force is applied with both the wrist and the thumb, enough to reach into the tissues.

As a rule, this method is done with one hand, or with both hands alternately. Both hands can also be used simultaneously, as shown in Diagram 11. Enough force should be applied to reach down to the vital energy. Tapping

---

8. *Pitu:* a line along the base of the thumb. See below, p. 71 and Diagram 61.
9. *Sanguan:* a line along the radial side of the forearm. See below, p. 71 and Diagram 61.

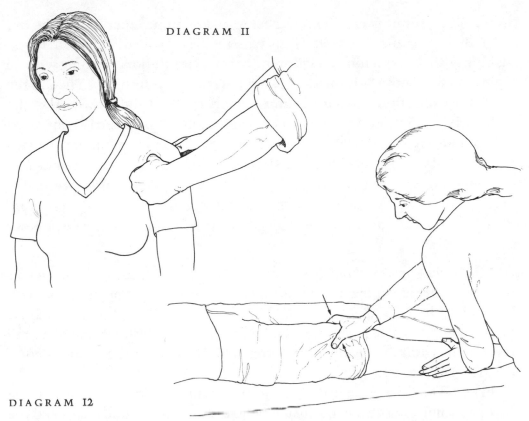

DIAGRAM II

DIAGRAM 12

the vital energy[10] is the main requirement for restoring a deficient, diseased body to health. Select the acupoints or pain-sites to be massaged, establish their locations precisely, and then proceed to apply the thumb-tip push to them one by one in a definite order. The thumb-tip moves quickly, making a rotating motion at the same time. This method is, therefore, also called the "tying-up method." This kind of technique is widely used clinically, with considerable success in tapping vital energy.

d) *Flat-Palm Push Method:* Push with the palm flat on the skin surface. The pushing is usually carried out from the farthest end of a limb towards the

---

10. Vital energy: *Qi (ch'i)*, the life-giving energy believed in Chinese traditional medicine to flow through the body in a system similar to the circulatory and nervous systems. Disturbance of the flow causes disease, and is relieved by acupuncture or massage of the acupoints. Most acupoints are located on meridians of the life-energy system.

trunk. When administered on the chest or abdomen, it must follow the rise and fall of breathing. Generally this method is divided into two types: pushing with an expiration and pushing to cause expiration. Pushing with an expiration does not start until the patient starts to breathe out. Then at the end of the expiration, the hand is immediately released and drawn back, and pushing is discontinued until the next expiration. This is carried out again and again in a repeated sequence. In pushing to cause expiration, the patient's breathing follows the pushing action. Pushing forcefully causes expiration, and releasing and withdrawing causes inspiration. The latter technique works well to improve function of the respiratory system, and therefore is applicable to the patient affected with incapacity of function of the respiratory system.

e) Palm-Heel Push Method: Push forcefully on the skin, using the muscular pads on either side of the heel of the hand. In the course of pushing forward, these muscular pads are used to pinch the area gradually tighter and tighter. (See Diagram 12.) The pushing generally goes from the farthest end of a limb towards the trunk, returning to the original position after the action is completed to begin again.

This kind of massage is usually done on the limbs, and is divided into the slow push and smooth push, depending on the amount of force used and the speed of the pushing. When the slow push is used, the speed is slower and there is less force. In the smooth push the speed is faster and there is greater force: after a swift push, the hand is at once withdrawn from the limb, brought back to the starting point, and the push is repeated. This procedure is repeated over and over again. The smooth push method can effectively reach down into the muscles and enhance muscular stimulation.

4. The Grasp Method

The grasp method is a type of massage that involves using the fingers to grasp and lift the muscle.

It is usually combined with acupoint massage. The grasping and lifting movements are done comparatively quickly. Applying the grasp to an area 2–3 times is usually sufficient. The amount of strength applied in grasping should result in the patient experiencing a feeling of soreness and swelling during massage, and after massage a loose easy feeling. If pain is felt, after the grasping, this shows that the force used was too great.

The grasping method is divided into three different ways: the three-finger grasp, five-finger grasp, and shaking grasp.

a) Three-Finger Grasp Method: To grasp with the thumb, index, and third fingers is sufficient for small areas, such as the *jianjing*[11] point on the shoulder (see Diagram 13), the *weizhong*[12] point at the back of the knee, and the back of the neck.

b) Five-Finger Grasp Method: This type of grasp uses the thumb and the four fingers, and is suitable for large, muscular areas, such as the front of the thigh (the musculus quadriceps femoris) and the back of the calf (the musculus gastrocnemius).

c) Shaking Grasp Method: After grasping with the fingers, do a light shaking, gradually allowing the fingers grasping the muscle to loosen. This is suitable for massage of the abdominal region.

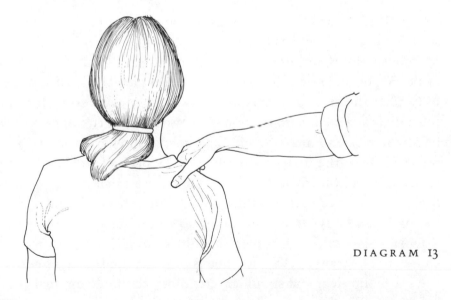

DIAGRAM 13

---

11. *Jianjing:* an acupoint at the highest point on the shoulder. See below, p. 67 and Diagram 59.
12. *Weizhong:* an acupoint in the back of the knee. See below, p. 70 and Diagram 60.

Note: The muscle-snapping method. This is a special type of massage technique. It is similar to the grasp method, but the manipulation is much stronger, and the degree of stimulation is greater. It is used with muscles such as the biceps and triceps of the arm and the outer hamstrings. With the thumb, index, and middle fingers, grasp the muscle by the intermuscular septum, either at its thickest point or near the muscle tendon, and draw it to one side. Having drawn it to a certain point, let it slip from between the fingers, like drawing a bow and shooting arrows. A snapping sound will then be heard and the patient will have a strong feeling of soreness and swelling, which is soon converted to a light, loose sensation.

The method can only be used on one muscle 1–2 times. It should be followed by some other methods of massage to relieve the strong stimulation and produce relaxation.

This method is suitable for injuries to the soft tissues and for rheumatic disorders, especially for muscular strains, rheumatic muscle pains, etc.

5. The Roll Method

The roll method is a form of massage where the back of the hand is rolled over the body. It can be done with one hand, with both hands alternately, or with both hands simultaneously. With the hand in a loose fist, use the side of the hypothenar pad along with the upper part of the fifth metacarpal joint to contact the area to be massaged. Press down with some force, while making a vigorous backward motion. At this moment the fingers should quickly be slightly spread apart to add force to the movement. The points of force must all lie in the metacarpal joints of the back of the hand. In this method many back-and-forth rolling movements are made, and the application of force must be even and rhythmic. The rolling hand should seem attached to the patient's body; it should not jump around or strike the patient.

During the rolling the hand should gradually keep moving forward, as shown in Diagram 14. This method is properly applied to larger areas, such as the back, hip, leg, and shoulder, etc. Since the force applied goes so deep, it is best used on the spots where the muscle and soft tissues are thick. Though this method can be used independently, it is generally combined with other techniques. For example, at the very beginning of the massage, the rub and the knead methods may be used, and the roll method can follow them.

DIAGRAM 14

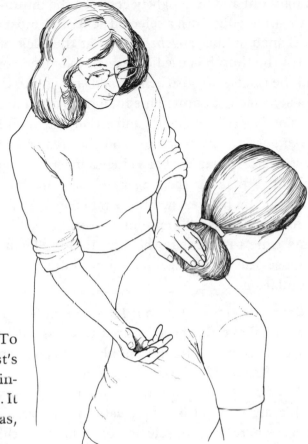

Note: Rolling Cylinder. To relieve the drain on a therapist's physical energy, a rolling cylinder made of wood can be used. It is suitable for broader areas, such as the back, thigh, etc.

6. The Dig Method

The dig method of massage involves a finger or fingers deeply digging into a certain part of the body or into a meridian point. It is also called the "finger-needle method." In massage therapy it is both unique and one of the most commonly used techniques. Where the dig method is performed, the practitioner has to trim his fingernails. The dig should be strong enough to result in the patient's feeling a sore swelling sensation.

The dig method is divided into the single-finger dig, bent-finger dig, and finger-cut methods.

a) Single-Finger Dig Method: The tip of the thumb or middle finger is used to press into the patient's flesh. When the middle finger is used, it is extended straight out and held tightly between the thumb and the index finger. The tip of the finger digs into a selected acupoint, most often one in the head or neck area, such as the *fengchi*[13] point at the back of the neck. (See Diagram 15.) When the thumb is used, the interphalangeal joint of the thumb is half bent, and the fingers are also bent to add strength to the dig. The thumb tip digs into a selected acupoint. This method is often used on the limbs, at acupoints such as *hegu*[14], *neiguan*[15] and *zusanli*[16]. In children, dig massage is applied at *neilaogong*[17], *yiwofeng*[18] and the greater and lesser *hengwen*[19].

No matter what kind of a single-finger dig is applied, force must be exerted gradually, making the finger-tip press in, but avoiding any sudden force. After the dig has reached the vital energy, that is when a flow of energy can be felt, continue to press for ½–1 minute. Vibration can be applied at the same time to intensify the stimulation. Then gradually relax the pressure and use the kneading method to soften the reaction resulting from the stimulation.

b) *Bent-Finger Dig Method:* First, the middle finger is bent. Then the first knuckle above the hand is used to press into the body. (See Diagram 16). During this procedure the thumb has to press against the last knuckle of the middle finger. The index and the fourth fingers are also bent, and the bent middle finger is pinched firmly into place, as shown in Diagram 16. The force of this dig method is very great, and it digs quite deeply. It is suitable for places where the muscle is comparatively thick. When the single-finger

---

13. *Fengchi:* acupoints located at the base of the skull, behind the ears. See p. 66 and Diagrams 57 and 59.
14. *Hegu:* an acupoint on the back of the hand, between the bones of the thumb and index finger. See p. 62 and Diagrams 57 and 59.
15. *Neiguan:* an acupoint on the underside of the forearm, above the wrist. See p. 62 and Diagrams 57 and 58.
16. *Zusanli:* an acupoint on the outer edge of the tibia, below the knee. See p. 68 and Diagram 60.
17. *Neilaogong:* an acupoint on the middle of the palm. See p. 70 and Diagram 61.
18. *Yiwofeng:* an acupoint on the back of the wrist. See p. 70 and Diagram 61.
19. Greater *hengwen*, lesser *hengwen:* acupoints in the fold of the wrist (greater) and in the folds at the bases of the fingers (lesser). See p. 70 and Diagram 61.

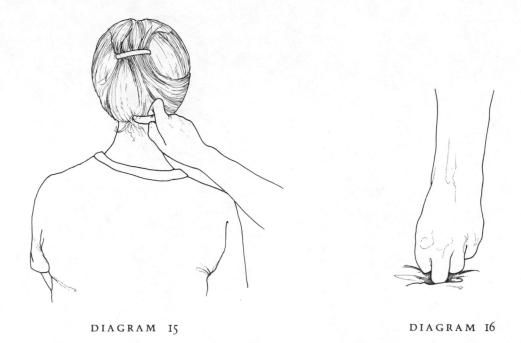

DIAGRAM 15   DIAGRAM 16

method fails to obtain a reaction, this method is usually found effective; for instance at such acupoints as *huantiao*,[20] *geshu*,[21] *ganshu*,[22] *pishu*,[23] and *weishu*,[24].

c) *The Finger-Cut method:* Use the end of the thumb to lightly and dexterously push along the skin in a dense pattern of strokes. (See Diagram 17.) As a rule this method is used only where the tissues are swollen. Since the swelling is pushed ahead of the finger, the movement must be toward the heart. Where a sprained joint is accompanied by swelling, this method can often cause the swelling to immediately disappear. The amount of force used must be small and the speed of stroke slow. Especially with any tender pressure point, be certain to avoid increasing the pain at the injured site.

---

20. *Huantiao:* an acupoint on the buttocks. See p. 67 and Diagram 59.
21. *Geshu:* an acupoint on the back, beside the lower end of the spinous process of the 7th thoracic vertebra. See p. 66 and Diagram 59.
22. *Ganshu:* near the 9th thoracic vertebra. See p. 66 and Diagram 59.
23. *Pishu:* near the 11th thoracic vertebra. See p. 66 and Diagram 59.
24. *Weishu:* near the 12th thoracic vertebra. See p. 67 and Diagram 59.

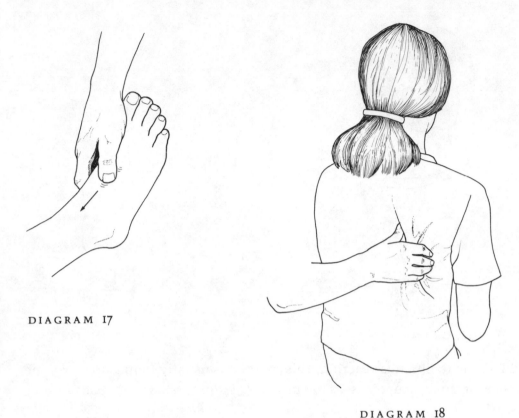

DIAGRAM 17

DIAGRAM 18

7. The Pluck Method

The pluck method is a type of massage which uses the hand to pluck at the muscles. It is also called the "pull method." This method is usually applied with one hand, using the side of the thumb and the tips of the index and third fingers to grasp the muscle at its tendinous portion and pluck with the appropriate amount of force. (See Diagram 18.) For instance, at the long and short origins of the biceps muscle of the arm, or the muscle on the inside edge of the scapula, this massage-method is applied 1–3 times, to the degree that the patient feels as much of a sore, swollen sensation as he can stand. This will produce a definite effect of relaxing muscle tension or freeing adhesion. There is also another type of pluck method, called the energy-system pluck method, which is very similar to this one.

8. The Kneading Method

The kneading method is a type of massage which involves making a kneading motion on the skin with the fingers or the palm. The palm and fingers are never withdrawn from contact with the skin, and the subcutaneous tissue in the area is allowed to slide along with them. Normally, this method is applied with one hand. The force used is relatively light, reaching only to the subcutaneous tissue. It has the effect of releasing the stimulation produced by stronger manipulations and of allaying pain. It is classified into the thumb kneading and palm kneading methods.

a) Thumb Kneading Method: The palmar surface of the thumb is pressed tightly against the skin and moved with a circular kneading motion. This method is suitable for restricted areas and acupoints. It is used in coordination with the single-finger dig massage to relieve the sore, swelling reaction that method gives rise to. The force used in kneading should be increased from light to heavy, and then decreased from heavy to light again.

b) Palm Kneading Method: With the heel of the palm, or the whole palm, pressing closely against the skin, knead with a rotating motion, going either clockwise or counterclockwise. This is appropriate for larger areas, such as the abdominal region (see Diagram 19), or the back. In the course of palm-kneading, though the palm does not shift position, the range of the sliding movement of the subcutaneous tissue is allowed to become wider and wider. Also the force applied gradually becomes heavier and heavier. The rate of frequency in the palm kneading method is generally slow, about 50–60 times per minute.

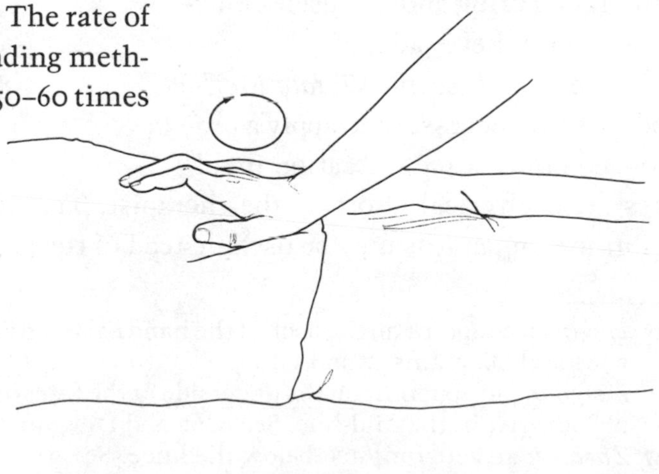

DIAGRAM 19

9. The Vibrate Method

This method uses a fingertip, or the palm, to apply vibration to a part of the body or to an acupoint. In this method, the practitioner's arm, especially the muscles of forearm and hand, must exert a strong static force that becomes concentrated at the fingertip, or in the palm, making the massaged area vibrate. It is important that the vibration rate be high, and that the force used be great. Most often, one hand is used, but two hands can also be used simultaneously. This method comprises the finger and palm vibrate techniques.

a) *Finger Vibrate Method:* Vibration is applied with the thumb or the middle finger to the tissue in the area to be massaged. The posture of the hand is similar to the one used in the single-finger dig method. This method is often used following the single-finger dig. It is employed to step up stimulation after the sore, swelling reaction produced by the dig method. Continue vibration for about ½–1 minute. The finger-vibrate method is also applied to such acupoints as *hegu*[25] (see Diagram 20), *neiguan*[26] and *zusanli*[27]. It is also used on acupoints in the abdominal region, but here it must always follow the rise and fall of breathing. Apply the pressure with expiration; release the pressure with inspiration.

b) *Palm Vibrate Method:* The vibration is applied with the flat surface of the palm pressed against the skin. This method is appropriate for larger areas such as the thigh, lower back, etc. It can bring about muscle-relaxation and relieve pain.

Note: The Electric Vibrate Method: As it is necessary to apply a prolonged static force, vibration invol-

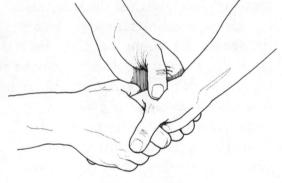

DIAGRAM 20

ves great physical effort by the therapist. To ease this burden, an electric vibratory apparatus may be used instead of the hand.

---

25. *Hegu:* an acupoint on the back of the hand between the thumb and index finger. See p. 62 and Diagrams 57 and 59.
26. *Neiguan:* an acupoint on the underside of the forearm, two inches above the crease of the wrist in the mid-line. See p. 62 and Diagrams 57 and 58.
27. *Zusanli:* an acupoint just below the knee. See p. 68 and Diagram 60.

10. The Drag Method

The drag method involves pressing down on the skin with the fingers and then drawing them to one side with steady pressure. It is generally done with the flats of both thumbs simultaneously. The special characteristic of this method is the use of even, sustained pressure and a slow, gradual movement.

For headache, this method can be combined with other massage methods. The thumbs are dragged apart from the *yintang*[28] acupoint between the eyebrows toward the *taiyang*[29] acupoints in the temples. (See Diagram 21.) Then they are either dragged along both sides of the head back to the *fengchi*[30] acupoints on either side of the base of the skull or to the *tinggong*[31] acupoints in front of the ears. Repeat two or three times. The patient usually feels his head and eyes become lighter and clearer than before. This method can also be used to reduce swelling.

The Muscle Straightening Method: This massage technique is similar to the drag method. The only difference between them is that the muscle-straightening method is done more forcefully, to reach down into the muscle. The flat of one or both thumbs (or of the thumb and index finger, or of the middle finger) is used. With an even and continuous pressure, follow the muscle direction from up to down, or from up diagonally down. The force exerted by the fingers, must be steady and their movement slow, and their force must not be relaxed during the movement. A tense muscle can be brought to complete relaxation by going down the muscle fibres several times.

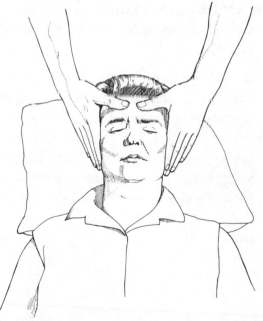

DIAGRAM 21

---

28. *Yintang:* See p. 60 and Diagram 58.
29. *Taiyang:* See p. 60 and Diagram 57.
30. *Fengchi:* See p. 66 and Diagrams 57 and 59.
31. *Tinggong:* See p. 60 and Diagram 57.

11. The Chafe Method

The chafe method is a type of massage which produces friction on the skin, using the fingers or the palm. The force used in this method must depend upon the reaction of the patient's skin. It is not desirable to exert too heavy a force. The purpose is just to reach as far as the skin and the subcutaneous tissue. The rate of speed of the movements is generally more than 100 times a minute. It is done with only one hand, and can be divided into two types, the finger chafe method and the palm-edge chafe method:

a) *The Finger Chafe Method:* This method involves rubbing the skin with the fingers. It is particularly useful for a paralyzed limb. When the finger-chafe method is applied to a paralyzed finger or toe, the practitioner holds the limb firmly in place with his left hand, fits the three middle fingers of his right hand around the affected finger or toe and chafes back and forth. In this way, the three sides of the finger can be rubbed simultaneously, as shown in Diagram 22.

b) *Palm-Edge Chafe Method:* The outer edge of the palm is used to chafe the skin. This method is often applied on either side of the back in cases of common cold, rheumatic pain, and gastroenteric disorders. The patient takes a sitting position, while the practitioner stands in front of him. This massage can be applied directly on the skin or through the clothing. Go up and down along both sides of the back with a fast sawing motion, continuing until the patient's skin becomes red. (See Diagram 23.)

DIAGRAM 22

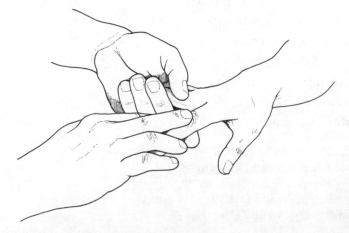

DIAGRAM 23

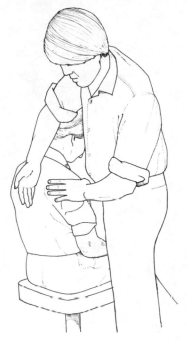

12. The Rub-Roll Method

The rub-roll method is a form of massage where the affected limb of the patient is taken between the two hands and rubbed with a rolling motion. It is suitable only for the limbs. The action of this massage can reach as far as the subcutaneous tissue, the muscle, and even the bones. During the course of massage, increase speed from slow to fast, then decrease it from fast to slow again. The method is divided into the palm rub-roll and palm-edge rub-roll methods:

a) Palm Rub-Roll: The left and right palms are placed on either side of the affected limb and rubbed back and forth. If the upper limb is to be rubbed, the patient should be seated, and the arm will naturally hang downward, as shown in Diagram 24. Or else, if sitting opposite the practitioner, the patient can rest his arm upon the practitioner's shoulder.

When the lower limb is to be rubbed, have the patient take a half-seated position and bend his knee. Or if the patient is lying on a bed, have the patient's leg rest on the practitioner's shoulder. In the case of the arm, the rub-rolling goes back and forth from shoulder to elbow and elbow to shoulder. With the lower limb the motion goes from knee to hip and hip to knee.

DIAGRAM 24

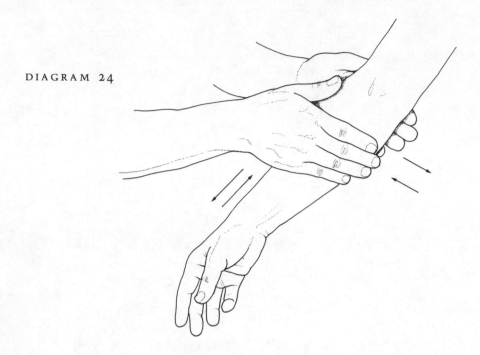

b) *Palm-edge Rub-Roll:* Apply the rub-roll with the outer edges of the palms on either side of the limb to be massaged. The body positions of both patient and therapist are similar to those in the palm rub-roll method. The effects of the palm-edge rub-roll can reach deeper into muscle, and the patient will experience a sore, swelling sensation.

13. The Pinch Method

The pinch method is a type of massage employing the fingers to squeeze and pinch muscle and ligamentous tissue. Pinch the flesh with the thumb on top and the rest of the fingers below and then roll the thumb and fingers over one another while moving forward, following the outline of the muscle. The right and left hands can be used alternately or simultaneously. The pinch method is divided into the three-finger pinch and the five-finger pinch.

a) *Three-Finger Pinch Method:* The thumb, forefinger, and middle finger are used. Pinch the muscle between the flats of the thumb and fingers and then use wrist-action to pinch and roll forward at the same time. This method is suitable for smaller areas, such as the fingers, palm, and forearm. (See Diagram 25.) In comparatively confined areas, the fingertips should be used to dig deep enough into the tissues for the massage to be effective.

DIAGRAM 25

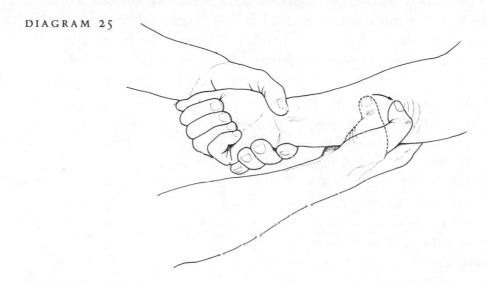

b) *Five Finger Pinch:* This process is performed with all five fingers. The method is similar to that of the three-finger pinch. It is best suited to larger areas such as the thigh, leg, shoulder, etc.

Note: Spinal Pinch Method: This method is often used with children. With the thumbs and forefingers of both hands, pinch the skin and sub-cutaneous tissues on either side of the spinal column. Release the skin and subcutaneous tissues as you move upward, alternating hands. Go from the buttocks up to the shoulder and neck areas (see Diagram 79).

14. The Tweak Method

The tweak method, also called the "twist method" is a form of massage using the thumb and index finger to pull up a part of the skin and subcutaneous tissues, and then quickly release them. In the course of this maneuver the hand holding the pinched tissue is made to turn slightly backwards, pulling the pinched tissues to one side, before quickly releasing them. (See Diagram 26). At this moment a snapping sound is often heard. Continue tweaking the same skin in the same direction until redness appears. In severe cases the skin can be tweaked until it develops red blotches.

Tweaking with one hand is suitable for the back, neck, and abdominal areas. This method is widespread among the Chinese people and has been transmitted from generation to generation. The common cold, headache, and gastro-intestinal upset all respond well to it. It can also be used in some pediatric diseases, such as normal common colds and fever, disturbed diges-tion, etc.

When the pinch method is ap-plied to children, generally both hands are used, and the palmar sur-faces of the thumb and forefinger are held together like pincers. After the skin is pinched and twisted, it is immediately and smoothly releas-ed. In this way the two hands tweak and release alternately until the skin begins to show redness.

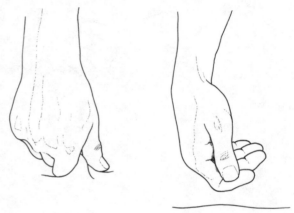

DIAGRAM 26

15. The Flick Method

The flick method is performed by using a finger to flick against the body. The index finger is bent against the thumb or middle finger, and then flicked forcefully against the body. The strength of the spring-like strikes should go from light to heavy, but never to a degree that would give rise to any pain. It can suitably to be applied to any joint, flicking the soft tissue around the joint. (See Diagram 27.) It can be used to treat aching joints.

16. The Knock Method

The knock method is a form of massage involving knocking on the tissue with the tips of the fingers. Force must be applied with both the wrist and the fingertips. The knocking must be dexterous, forceful, and elastic, and at

DIAGRAM 27

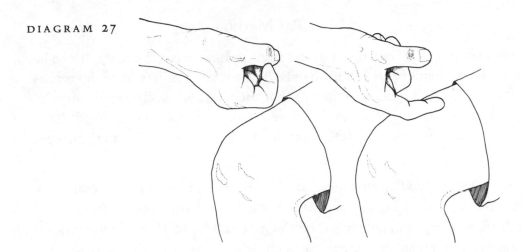

the same time a conscious rhythm must be maintained. The knocking method gives rise to an oscillating force that can reach down to the bone. It is divided into the middle-finger knock and five-finger knock method:

a) *Middle-Finger Knock Method:* For this method the middle finger is half-bent, and the wrist is relaxed. The knocking then proceeds with a bend-extend motion. This method is appropriate for use all around the scalp area.

b) *Five-Finger Knock Method*: In this method the five fingers are drawn close to one another, the fingertips are held even with each other, and the wrist is relaxed. In order to carry out the knocking the fingers are repeatedly bent and extended. They strike the body in the same way that a chicken pecks grain. For this reason it is also called "the peck method." It is appropriate for use on all parts of the forehead. (Diagram 28.)

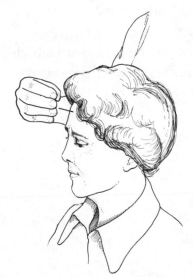

DIAGRAM 28

17. The Pat Method

The pat method uses the fingers or the palm to lightly pat the body. It can be done with one hand or with both hands. The movement has to be dexterous and elastic. For this reason it requires that the wrist be exceptionally supple. When both hands are used, their movements must be co-ordinated. This method is classified into the finger pat, back-of-the-fingers pat, and palm pat methods.

a) Finger Pat Method: In this method, the fingers and thumb are spread wide apart. The fingers are slightly bent, and the palmar surfaces of the fingers and thumb are employed to lightly pat on the patient's body. (See Diagram 29.) It is appropriate for use on the back and chest areas, and is often used in the massage of children.

b) Back-of-the-Fingers Pat Method: Here the fingers are slightly spread apart, and the finger joints are slightly bent. The index, middle, ring, and little fingers are used to vigorously pat the body, as shown in Diagram 30. This method is suitable for the limbs and can also be used on the chest and back areas.

c) Palm Pat Method: Here the center of the palm has to be raised by flexing the metacarpal joints, and the fingers drawn close together, leaving a hollow in the palm with which to pat the body. This method is suitable for the back area.

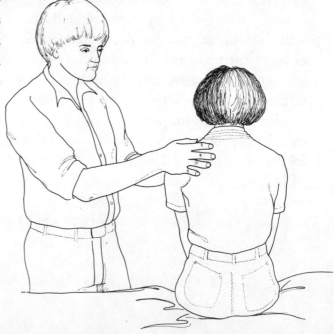

DIAGRAM 29

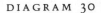

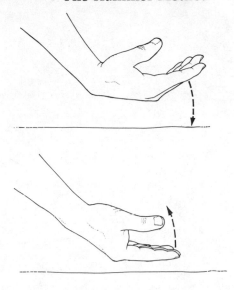

18. The Hammer Method

This is a type of massage which uses the fist to hammer on the body. The force used is heavier than that of the pat method and goes deeper into the muscles, joints, and bones. In this method the principal force comes from the wrist. Co-ordination and dexterity are required. The force used should be increased from light to heavy, while at the same time the blows remain elastic. The rate of speed is increased from slow to fast, or alternates between periods of slow and fast strokes. As a rule both hands are used simultaneously. This method is divided into the prone-fist hammer, upright-fist hammer, and palm-edge hammer methods, as follows:

a) Prone-Fist Hammer Method: Here both hands are held in loosely-clenched fists. The second knuckles of the four fingers are all held even with each other, and used to exert a hammering force on the body. This method is appropriate for areas where there is fleshy, thick muscle, such as the thigh area.

b) Upright-Fist Hammer Method: Here both hands are formed into clenched fists, with the fingers slightly spread apart. The thumb is bent and wrapped in the fist, or nests between the index and middle fingers. The fist is turned thumb upward, and the body is hammered with the fleshy part of the fist on the outer side of the palm. (See Diagram 31.) This method is suitable for the joint areas.

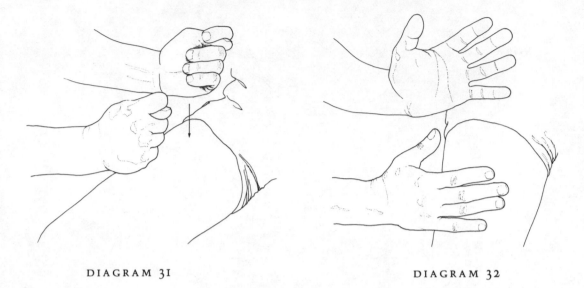

DIAGRAM 31   DIAGRAM 32

c) Palm-Edge Hammer Method: Here the fingers of both hands are extended and spread apart. The hammer massage is applied with the outer edge of the hand, as shown in Diagram 32. The method is appropriate for fleshy, muscular areas such as the thigh or the back.

Note: In order both to avoid tiring the therapist and to make the massage more comfortable for the patient, the hammering can be carried out with a mallet made from a piece of sponge rubber attached to a bamboo stick. Use two of these mallets, one in each hand.

19. The Extension Method

The extension method is a form of massage which helps a malfunctioning joint to regain its normal extension. This technique can be classified as a form of passive manipulation. In this method the extent to which the affected joint can be moved must first be carefully tested. Then a slow, even, continuous force is applied to bring about the appropriate amount of extension. In general, this should not cause the patient any pain. A sudden force or violent extension must never be used. Before each treatment the amount of increased movement that is possible for the affected joint must be carefully estimated. The range of extension is gradually increased. For the manipulation, the practitioner and the patient must be properly and securely positioned. The most frequently-used techniques are the shoulder-extension and elbow-extension methods.

a) Shoulder-Extension Method: In this method the patient takes a sitting position, while the practitioner stands in a half-crouch beside him, with his legs astride in the rider's position.[32] The affected limb rests on the back of the practitioner's neck, with the elbow resting on the practitioner's shoulder. The practitioner's hands are cupped over the patient's shoulder. (See Diagram 33.) The practitioner then slowly stands up, causing the patient's shoulder to abduct and bend forward to the appropriate extent. Maintain a fixed height for about 2–3 minutes before allowing the patient's shoulder to fall back. After a short pause the extension is repeated. The height of the second stretch may be slightly increased, but this must not be forced. The process should be repeated 3–5 times.

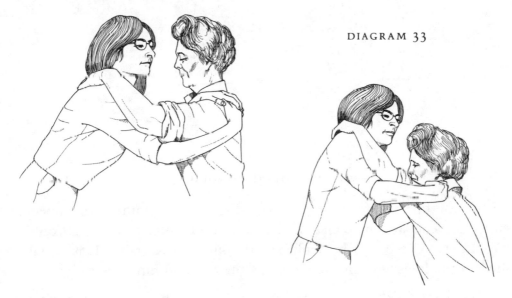

DIAGRAM 33

b) Elbow-Extension Method: In this method the patient sits opposite the practitioner. The practitioner cups the elbow of the affected arm, while the hand of the affected arm is pinned in the practitioner's armpit. The practitioner's other hand is placed on top of the affected shoulder. (See Diagram 34.) Then while pushing on the shoulder, he lifts up the patient's elbow, extending the joint. The degree of force used and amount of extension will depend upon the individual case, but violent force must be avoided.

---

32. Rider's position: legs spread apart and crouching slightly, as if riding a horse.

DIAGRAM 34

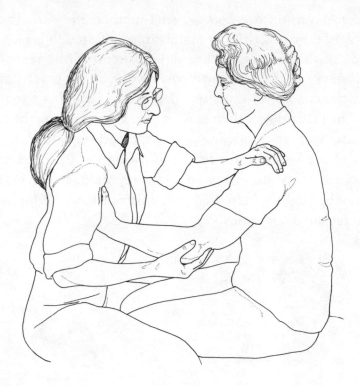

20. The Bend Method

The bend method is a form of massage which helps a joint with impeded mobility to bend. It can be classified as a form of passive manipulation. In this method, force has to be applied with skill and restraint. It is usually applied to the lower extremities, such as the calf and hip.

a) *Calf-Bend Method:* Here the patient lies face down, and the practitioner stands beside him, on the side of the affected limb. The practitioner grasps the affected calf with one hand, while the other holds the sole of the patient's foot. Then the knee joint is gradually bent. (See Diagram 35.) The movements begin slowly, but gradually become faster. The extent of the bending must correspond with the degree of movement possible for the joint.

b) *Hip-Bend Method:* Here the patient lies on his/her back, while the practitioner stands beside the affected limb. One hand holds the patient's kneecap, while the other grasps the sole of the foot, and the hip, knee, and

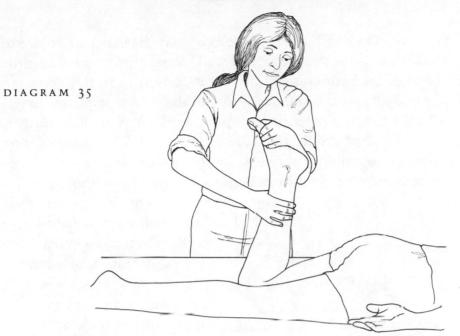

DIAGRAM 35

ankle are all made to bend at the same time. The practitioner then exerts a downward force to help the bending, the patient also tending actively to bend the limb. The thigh should be brought as close to the body as possible. (See Diagram 36.) The extent of the bending must correspond with the degree of movement possible for the joint.

c) *Two-hip Bend Method:* In this method the patient lies on his/her back, while the practitioner grasps the soles of the patient's feet with one hand, and with the other holds the kneecap area. The practitioner bends the knees and hips to a certain limit, and then elastically and rhythmically pushes

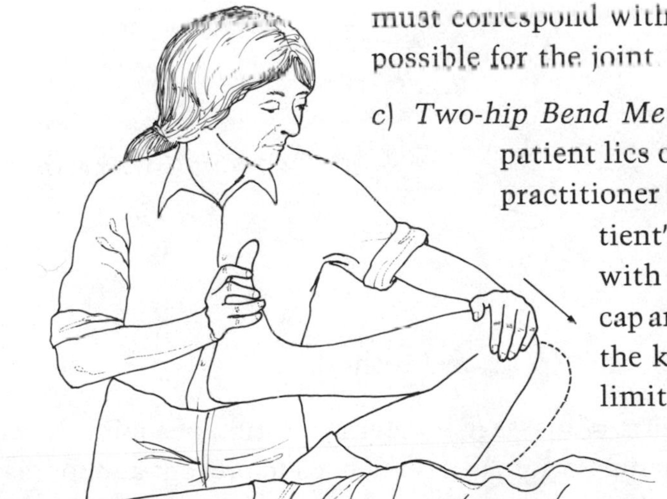

DIAGRAM 36

forward. The extent to which the hips are bent may gradually be enlarged, bringing the thigh close to the abdominal wall. Next, the hand holding the feet is switched to the buttocks, and the whole body is bent. (Diagram 37.) Care must be taken to progress gradually and in the correct sequence, in accordance with the patient's potential mobility. As the hips are bent further, the amount of force used should gradually be increased. This manipulation not only promotes the mobility of the hip joint but also improves the ability of the spinal column to bend forward. Because of this, the method is appropriate in some cases of chronic low back pain and arthritic stiffness. In addition, it can be selectively applied in the case of protrusion of a lumbar intervertebral disk, where it can promote the return to its proper position of the area of the slipped disk.

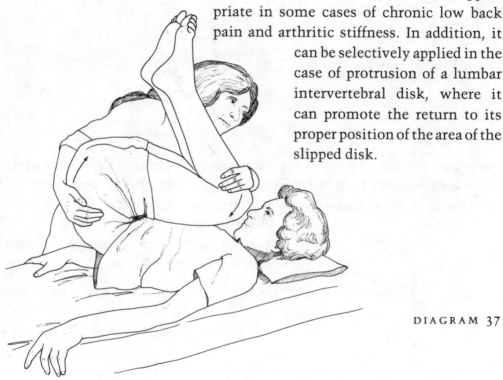

DIAGRAM 37

21. The Rotation Method

The rotation method is a form of massage involving rotation of a joint. It can be classified as a passive manipulation. It is often used to prevent and to treat functional disturbances of the rotatory movement of a joint. This method is applied to joints of all sizes from the knuckle joints to those as large as the joints in the lumbar and hip areas. Before applying this procedure, it is necessary to be familiar with the range of physiological movement in each joint and to observe in detail the state of joint mobility resulting from a disease. The direction of rotation is generally clockwise, and the speed should be slow rather than fast. The procedure for rotating the small joints in the hand, etc., is relatively simple. But when applying rotation to large joints, the patient has to be placed in a specific position.

The method is divided into the neck rotation, shoulder rotation, hip rotation and lumbar rotation methods.

a) Neck Rotation Method: The patient takes a sitting position and the therapist stands behind him. He places one hand under the patient's jaw and the other on the top of his head, slowly swinging the neck from one side to the other with his hands. When the muscles are relaxed, and the neck is turned completely to one side, the therapist takes advantage of its tendency to turn back in the opposite direction and gives it a sudden and forceful twist in that opposite direction, though not more than 90° in extent (See Diagram 38.) This method should be applied only once at a time, and not repeated. After the neck has been twisted, the patient usually feels it suddenly more flexible and comfortable. This method is always used in torticollis (stiff neck).

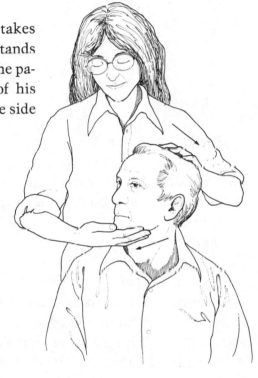

DIAGRAM 38

b) Shoulder Rotation Method, type I: The patient takes a sitting position. The practitioner stands firmly beside him with legs spread apart in the archer's position.[33] He grasps the patient's palm with one hand and holds his wrist with the other. First the patient's upper arm is pulled straight, then it is rotated. In the course of this rotation, the practitioner's hands must alternate with each other in holding the wrist area, never letting go. (See Diagram 39.)

33. Archer's position: Legs spread apart, one forward and one back, as if about to shoot with a bow and arrow.

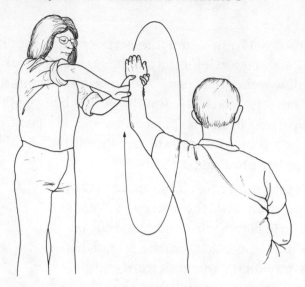

DIAGRAM 39

Shoulder Rotation Method, type 2: The patient sits with the elbow of the affected limb bent. The practitioner uses his own forearm and hand to support and hold the forearm of the affected arm, while his other hand presses on the patient's shoulder. He then rotates the shoulder clockwise and counter-clockwise.

Shoulder Rotation Method, type 3: The patient is seated with the affected arm relaxed and held out to one side. The practitioner grasps the hand of the affected arm with his own hand on the same side (i.e. his right hand for the patient's right hand, or vice-versa). He then turns the arm clockwise and counterclockwise. (See Diagram 40.) The rotation should be deft and vigorous like spinning cotton into yarn.

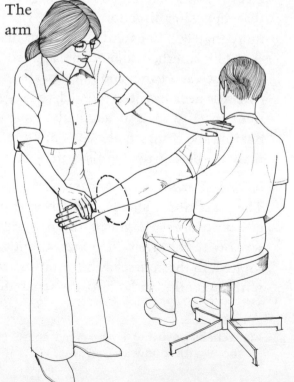

DIAGRAM 40

DIAGRAM 41

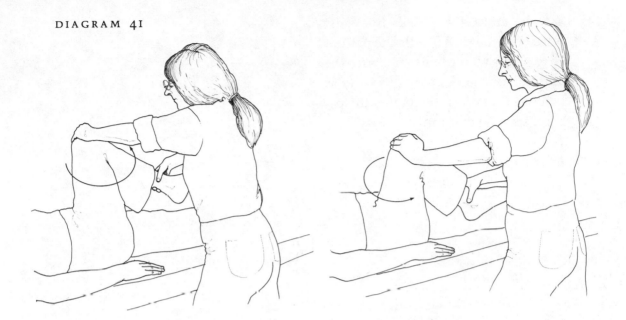

c) Hip Rotation Method: The patient lies on his back, with the therapist standing beside him. With one hand the therapist supports the patient's kneecap, and with the other grasps his calf, a third of the way up from the ankle. The hip and knee joints are half bent, and then the hip joint is rotated alternately clockwise and counterclockwise. (Diagram 41.)

d) Lumbar Rotation Method: In lumbar rotation, the therapist must stand firmly, shifting his center of gravity to follow the direction of the rotation. He must also be quite strong. If he is not strong, the range of the rotation he applies should not be too great, or he may lose his balance and fall.

Lumbar Rotation Method, type 1: The patient is seated while the therapist stands beside him with his legs apart, or in front of him with his legs astride. One hand is passed under the patient's armpit and grasps the opposite shoulder; the other reaches across the abdomen to hold the farther side of the waist. Then the patient is told to relax his whole body and the spine is rotated. (See Diagram 42.)

Lumbar Rotation Method, type 2: The patient is told to stand facing a crossbar, or the back of a steady chair. He graps the crossbar with both hands and bends his body slightly forward. The therapist stands behind him, legs

astride, and tightly holds his waist
with both hands. He tells the patient
to relax his whole body and, with the
vertical axis of the patient's body as
center of rotation, he rotates the patient's spinal column.

DIAGRAM 42

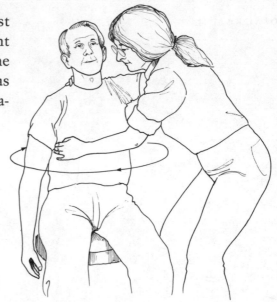

22. The Shake Method

This method is a form of massage that involves shaking the limbs, and can
be classified as a passive manipulation. It is applied only to the upper and
lower limbs. The practitioner holds the end of the patient's limb and shakes
it gently like a rope, making it rise and fall in waves. The method is classified
into two types, the upper-limb shake and lower-limb shake methods.

a) *Upper-Limb Shake Method, type* 1: The patient has to be seated, while
the practitioner stands on one side of him. Using both hands to hold the five
fingers of the affected limb and pull the limb tight, the practitioner moves
the limb with a shaking motion. The range of the shaking is increased from
small to large, so that waves are transmitted all the way to the shoulder.
This shaking movement is performed 3–5 times.

   Upper-Limb Shake, type 2: The patient is in either a sitting or a standing
position, while the therapist stands beside him. The patient's shoulder is
held firmly with one hand and the hand of the affected limb is grasped with
the other. The affected limb is then pulled out tight and shaken up and down
or left and right. (See Diagram 43.)

b) *Lower-Limb Shake Method:* The patient lies on his side and the therapist stands behind his feet. The therapist grasps the toes and back of the foot of the affected leg with his two hands, lifts the leg and shakes it. This is repeated 3–5 times.

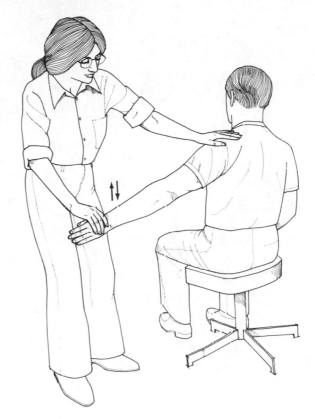

DIAGRAM 43

23. The Stretch Method

The stretch method is a type of massage which stretches the joints. It is a special form of passive manipulation. The pulling motion must be dexterous but forceful. The method has the functions of stretching contracted muscles and helping to restore a joint to its proper position. It may be divided into the following forms:

a) *Lumbar Stretch Method, type* I: The patient lies on his side, affected side upward, and the practitioner stands behind his back. The thumb of one hand is used to press on the painful part of the lumbus, while the other forearm supports the calf of the affected leg, with the hand cupping the kneecap. After bending the thigh upward toward the abdomen a few times, deftly and forcefully pull the leg out backwards. At the same time, the thumb pushing against the aching area exerts a little extra pressure. (See Diagram 44.) This process is repeated 5–6 times. This method is suitable in cases of slipped

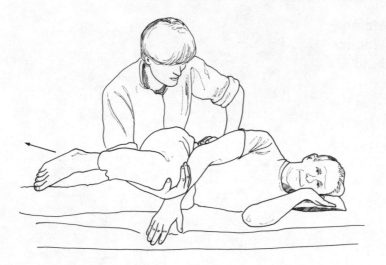

DIAGRAM 44

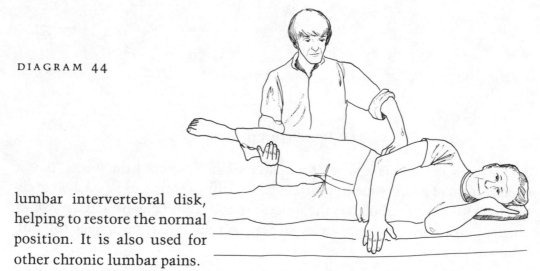

lumbar intervertebral disk, helping to restore the normal position. It is also used for other chronic lumbar pains.

Lumbar Stretch Method, type 2: Practitioner and patient stand back to back. The practitioner uses his elbows to hook the patient's arms and lifts the patient up so that the practitioner's buttocks are somewhat lower than the patient's. Then the patient is told to relax his whole body. The practitioner bends and straightens his knees repeatedly, forcefully shaking the patient with his buttocks, thereby stretching the patient's spinal column. (See Diagram 45.) To finish up, the practitioner can swing the patient's body from side to side several times.

DIAGRAM 45

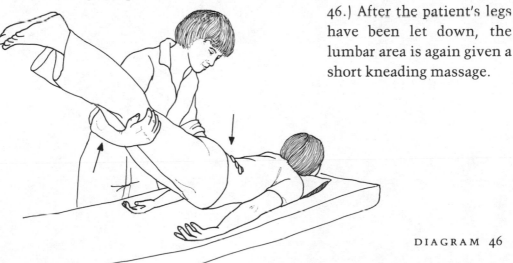

Lumbar Stretch Method, type 3: Here the patient lies face down. The practitioner first uses the kneading and rub methods to relax the muscles of the lumbar area. Then he places his forearms under the patient's kneecaps and lifts the lower half of the patient's body so that only the chest is touching the bed. He places his other hand on the patient's lower lumbar region and presses and releases several times in a rhythmic and elastic manner. When the patient's muscles have become quite relaxed, the practitioner suddenly uses his forearm to press down hard on the patient's lumbar area. Simultaneously, the forearm which is supporting the patient's knees is raised upward with force, causing the patient's lumbar area to extend backward. (See Diagram 46.) After the patient's legs have been let down, the lumbar area is again given a short kneading massage.

DIAGRAM 46

Lumbar Stretch Method, type 4: Here the patient lies on his side with the affected side upward. The practitioner grasps the ankle of the leg on the affected side with his hands, and pulls the leg backward. At the same time he lifts his leg and places the sole of his foot tightly against the small of the patient's back simultaneously pulling with his hands and pushing with his foot. First, push lightly several times until you feel the patient's lumbar area has become comparatively relaxed. Then perform the combined pushing and pulling movement with a sudden, powerful force, causing the patient's lumbar region to extend backwards. (See Diagram 47.) Providing that an effective amount of strength is used, one such action is generally enough.

DIAGRAM 47

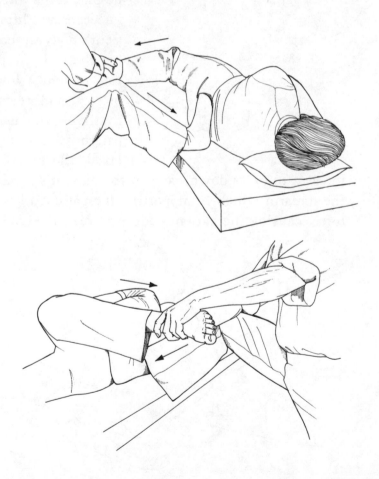

b) Upper-Limb Stretch: The patient sits on a low stool and the therapist stands facing him, a little towards the affected side. The affected arm is held out with the back of the hand toward the therapist, who grasps the fingers in two groups with his two hands. He rotates the arm in a circle from top inside to top outside, down and around again, several times. When the muscles of the affected limb feel as if they have relaxed, and the limb moves freely, the therapist suddenly and forcefully lifts it upward. (See Diagram 48.) This method has been found effective in treating patients with soreness in the upper limb or shoulder, but where movement of the joints is not greatly impeded. It is generally applied following the application of other methods of massage, and is used only once or twice at a time.

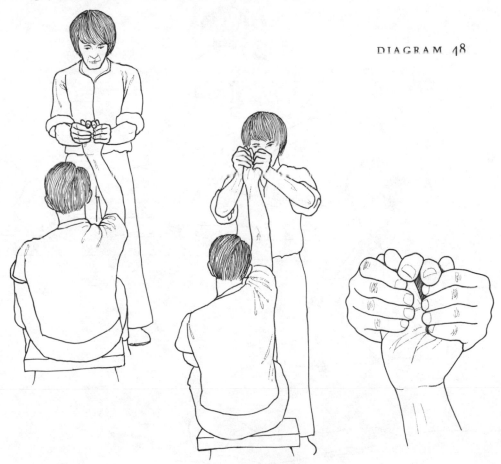

DIAGRAM 48

c) Lower-Limb Stretch Method: This method is also called moving the leg. The patient lies on his back. The practitioner supports the calf of the affected leg with one arm and hand, pressing the kneecap with the other hand. First the hip and knee joints are bent, and a slight amount of force is used to press the thigh downward. As soon as the thigh comes close to the abdominal area, the affected limb is dexterously and forcefully pulled out straight. At this point, with the hip joint half bent and the knee joint completely extended, the patient is told to kick his leg up and forward. (See Diagram 49.) The degree of bending of the hip joint must correspond with the height that the patient can raise a straight leg and the degree of elevation should gradually be increased. The movement is done 10–20 times during each session.

DIAGRAM 49

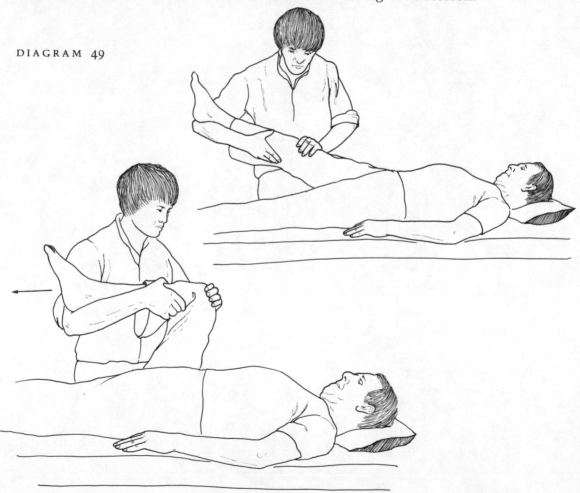

24. The Tread Method

The tread method is a form of massage involving treading on the patient's body. It is often applied to the lumbar area. The patient lies face down on a rather short massage bed. The pectoral area and the thigh each are cushioned with a pillow about 30 centimeters high, so that the lumbar region itself rests over empty space. The practitioner hangs tightly with his hands onto a sturdy bar fixed above the patient's bed. He lightly steps down on the lumbar-sacral area with one foot, first applying light pressure several times, then gradually increasing the force. He rhythmically alternates stepping down on the spine and releasing the pressure, rising and falling like the carrying-pole of someone carrying heavy loads on each shoulder. (See Diagram 50.) The patient is told to keep his mouth open and breathe in and out with the rhythm. The force of the treading is increased from light to heavy until an effective strength is reached. The treading is repeated about 20 times, then a rest, then treading again. Three to four bouts of treading can be done at one session. This method has the effect of hastening the restoration of a protruding intervertebral disk to its proper position.

DIAGRAM 50

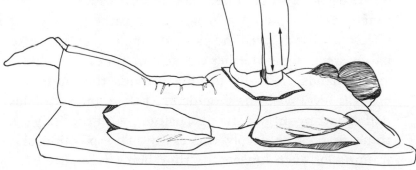

Section 2: Practicing Massage Techniques

Well-practiced technique, agile and flexible joints, and strong fingers are all necessary for massage therapy. The therapist's movements must be smooth, dexterous, and gentle, and he or she must be able to keep them up over long periods of time. Only under all these conditions can a good therapeutic effect be obtained. Consequently, it is necessary that the therapist undertake continuous training, building up his or her strength, and practicing the massage techniques, in order to serve the people better. Basically, training is divided into two parts: general physical training and practicing the finger-techniques.

1. Physical Training

Massage therapy calls for great physical strength, and especially for stamina. At the same time the practitioner must be able to maintain definite positions for long periods of time, such as standing with the legs spread apart in the rider's position or the archer's position (see Diagram 53, following). All this demands that the practitioner regularly engage in a good exercise program. The following introduces several exercises aimed at developing the strength of the limbs and the lumbar area.

Exercise 1: Stand with the feet shoulder-width apart. Hold the body erect, with the head slightly bent and the eyes looking straight ahead. Press the tongue against the upper palate and breathe through the nose. Then evenly raise both hands with the palms facing downward. After a deep breath, the palms are brought together and held in front of the chest, the fingertips of the joined hands gradually turning towards the chest, and the elbows being brought level with the shoulders. At the same time, flex the knees slightly, half squatting into the rider's position, with the body's gravity centred. Continue to breathe deeply and easily. This position should be held for 1–3 minutes or even longer, the time being gradually extended with practice. (See Diagram 51.)

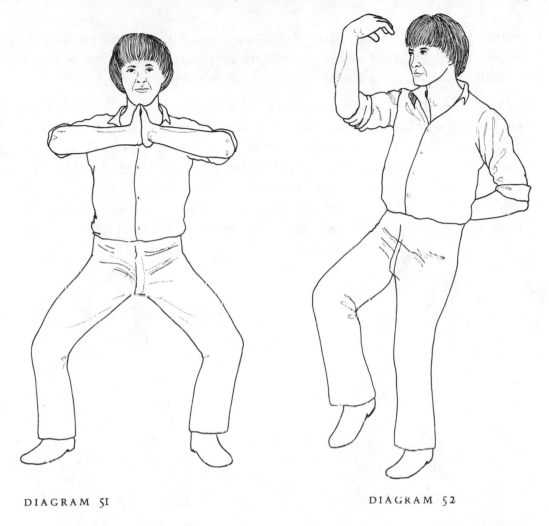

DIAGRAM 51   DIAGRAM 52

Exercise 2: After the first exercise has been completed, revert to a natural position and rest for a moment, then do Exercise 2. Take a half step forward with right foot and bend the left knee slightly, going into a half-crouch. The tip of the right foot touches the ground, and the heel is raised; the weight of the body is placed on the left leg. At the same time form the left hand into a loose fist and, with the center of the fist facing outward, place it behind the back. The five fingers of the right hand are extended straight and held closely together; the wrist is fully bent and rotated inward as far as it will go. The elbow forms a 90 degree angle and the upper arm is extended forward, level with the shoulder. Fix your eyes on your right hand, compose yourself, and breathe deeply. Hold this position for 1–3 minutes. Alternate the positions of the left and right hands and feet. (See Diagram 52.) In succeeding sessions, gradually increase the amount of time for which the position is held.

Exercise 3: After completing Exercise 2, relax and move freely, then do Exercise 3. Put the right foot forward in the archer's position, with the toes pointing forward. (See Diagram 53.) The left leg is extended backward, with the foot pointing to the side. The heels must be flat on the ground and planted firmly and the body erect, with its weight centered. A fist is made with the right hand and the wrist is bent and rotated inward as much as possible. The elbow area is bent at an obtuse angle and the upper arm held level with the

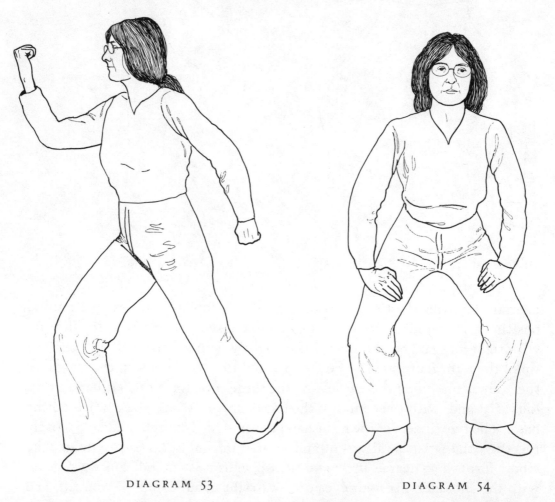

DIAGRAM 53   DIAGRAM 54

shoulder. Then, form the left hand into a fist, with the wrist bent. The elbow is slightly bent and the arm extended out behind the back. The head turns somewhat to the right, with the eyes on the right hand. Pull tightly with the right hand, like a cowherd holding a tight lead on a cow. Then take a deep, easy breath. This posture should be held for a certain length of time. The process is alternated, left and right, and the length of time for which it is held is gradually increased, with increasing ability.

Exercise 4: After completing Exercise 3, rest a while, then do Exercise 4. Set the legs shoulder-width apart, and gradually squat down until the knees are bent to about 90 degrees. Rest the hands on the legs above the kneecaps, with the thumbs on the outside of the kneecaps, so that the arms form a rough circle. Hold the chest area upright, and keep the weight of the body centered. Then, with the eyes looking straight ahead, do a deep-breathing exercise. This posture should be held for as long a period of time as possible, the longer the better. (See Diagram 54.)

After completing these four exercises, do some movements to relax.

2. Practicing the Techniques

Massage therapy is applied chiefly with the hands. Therefore, the hands must be trained to be strong, gentle, dexterous, well-coordinated, and untiring. The hand exercises are in two stages. The first stage involves practicing on a bag filled with sand. After becoming skillful with practice on the sandbag, then practice on the human body (two people can practice on each other). The sandbag may be sewn out of white linen or cotton cloth. The specifications for the sandbag are: one foot long, one foot wide, 2 inches high, and filled with cleanly-washed sand. The most commonly used massage techniques and the most important aspects of the practice are introduced below:

a) *The Thumb Push Method:* The thumb push is divided into three types: the flat-thumb push, side-of-the-thumb push, and thumb-tip push. However, the main aspects of practicing all of these are identical. In practicing the push method, a standing position is normal but a sitting position can also be used. Concentrate your thoughts; let the shoulders sink and the elbows hang down; flex the elbow; bend the wrist and let the hand hang down. The hand is held in a partial fist, with the fingers not allowed to go beyond the center of the palm. The thumb is extended and rests on the second knuckle joint of the index finger, covering the eye of the fist.[34] Now, with the tip of the thumb against the sandbag, swing from the wrist and move the thumb back and forth rhythmically so that the thumb is pushed out forward and then drawn back. (See Diagram 55.) In pushing out about two-thirds of one's strength is used, and in drawing back about one-third. When pushing forward, do not let the thumb jump, and in drawing back, do not let the bent phalangeal joint touch the surface of the sandbag. The thumb should push forward along a straight, and not an oblique line. The wrist should be completely relaxed. The rate of pushing is maintained at 120–160 times a minute. When this technique is perfected, the thumb will seem to be attached to the surface of the sandbag, attaining the requirement of: "Heavy but not rigid, light but not floating." It is best to perfect the use of both right and left hands, so that one hand can alternate with the other when this method is used clinically.

DIAGRAM 55

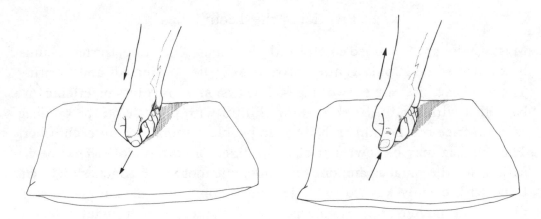

b) *The Roll Method:* Take a standing position; allow the shoulders to sink, and the elbows to hang down. One elbow is bent and the wrist relaxed; the hand is formed into a loose fist, with the center of the palm turned upward.

---

34. Eye of the fist: the index-finger end of a fist, the space in the crook of the finger is like an eye.

The fingers and thumb are somewhat bent, but not stiff; the index and middle fingers are extended freely. With the back of the fifth finger, together with the hypothenar pad, against the sandbag, make a backward-rolling motion with the wrist. Repeat this rolling exercise over and over again. (See Diagram 56.) Be careful to avoid making jumping movements, or any scraping, in order to prevent damage to the skin. Both hands must be trained to do the rolling smoothly, with deep-reaching force and unflagging rhythm, so that the hands can be alternated.

DIAGRAM 56

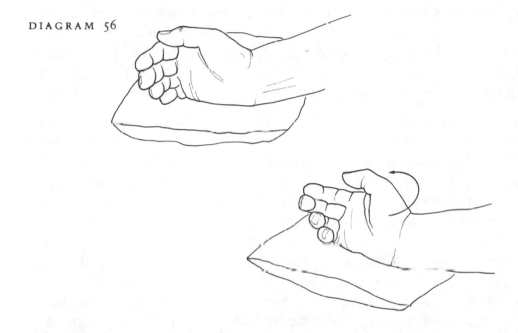

c) *The Finger-Vibrate Method:* The finger-vibrate method is applied with either the middle finger or the thumb, and generally with the right hand. In practicing the middle-finger vibration, the thumb and the index finger are used to hold the middle finger, and the tip of the middle finger is placed against the sandbag. In the thumb vibration, the outer edge of the thumb-tip contacts the sandbag. The wrist area is bent slightly toward the palm. Both the hand and the forearm muscles exert a static, tense force to produce a vibrating motion. It is possible that when one starts to practice, one may not be able to produce any vibration, or to sustain vibration for any length of time. But after some practice, vibration will be produced. The vibration should be slight and even, with the force coming from the tip of the finger. One should be able to sustain vibration for over a minute.

d) *The Pinch Method:* The pinch method most often uses the thumb, index, and middle fingers, and is usually done with one hand. It can be practiced along the edge of the sandbag. The thumb, index and middle fingers pinch together on the edge of the sandbag with a relatively strong force. At the same time the thumb moves clockwise with a rolling, rubbing, pinching motion. The index and middle fingers make a similar motion in the opposite direction. In the course of this rolling, rubbing, pinching motion, the fingers should gradually move forward. This technique calls for coordination, smoothness, sensitivity, and control of the amount of force imparted by the fingertips. One must be able to sustain it for over ten minutes at a time.

e) *The Hammer and Pat Methods:* Here both hands are usually used simultaneously. Whether the flats of the fingers are used for patting or the fist is used to hammer, the main aspects of the practice are the same. The surface of the hand used in hammering or patting must always make a flat contact. In patting, the flat of the fingers is used, and in hammering, a loose fist must be used. In patting the fingers are slightly bent and spread apart. In both hammering and patting, most of the movement should come from the wrist being swung up and down. The wrists should be trained to the point that they move smoothly and dexterously, but with strength. They should rise and fall in co-ordination, with an even rhythm. You should be able to change the rate of movement and sustain it for more than ten minutes at a time.

Practicing is often quite boring, especially at the beginning when you are likely to experience soreness, swelling, and fatigue. For this reason, your attitude must be serious, and you must be perservering and not lax. Moreover, as this sort of practice is also a form of physical exercise, it should be carried out according to the general rules of physical exercise. The following points are set forth for reference:
(i) Practice is best carried out early in the morning, after getting up, and in an open yard, or park.

(ii) During practice wear loose clothes and a loose belt. Do not wear clothing that is either too tight or too heavy.

(iii) Do not begin practicing when you are too full or too hungry. Generally, practice should not be done within 1½ hours after a meal.

(iv) Before the practice do some prepatory exercises: move your hands and your feet, and take a few deep breaths before beginning the practice session. Before practicing finger techniques, all the joints of the fingers should be flexed a bit.

(v) After the practice session, do some settling-down movements and deep breathing. If you have perspired, immediately rub yourself dry, and put on all your clothing.

(vi) During practice you have to concentrate your thoughts, in order to develop the good habit of devoting all your attention to carrying out the treatment. In this way, the practice sessions will achieve a greater effect and value, and you will be less likely to injure yourself.

(vii) In practicing the techniques, be aware of cleanliness and avoid scrapes and scratches. If the skin reacts sensitively, practice should be suspended.

CHAPTER III

ACUPOINTS COMMONLY USED IN MASSAGE THERAPY

Acupoints for Adults

Baihui: (acupoint on the governor vessel meridian) located on the midline at the top of the skull where it intersects with a line drawn connecting the tips of the left and right ears.

Yintang: (irregular acupoint not on a meridian) between the inner ends of the eyebrows, at the most prominent point of the frontal bone.

Taiyang: (irregular acupoint not on a meridian) in the depression about a finger's-width outside a point between the outer canthus of the eye and the tip of the eyebrow.

Jingming: (foot greater *yang*, bladder meridian) in the depression 1 *fen*[1] inside and above the inner canthus of the eye.

Zuanzhu: (foot greater *yang*, bladder meridian) in the depression at the inner end of the eyebrow, 1 *cun* from the median line.

Sibai: (foot bright *yang*, stomach meridian) in the depression just above the infraorbital foramen, 3 *fen* below the lower edge of the bony orbit.

Tinggong: (hand greater *yang*, small intestine meridian) in a depression in front of the tragus of the ear. Find the point when the mouth is open.

Tinghui: (foot lesser *yang*, gallbladder meridian) in a depression in front of the intertragic notch. Find the point when the mouth is open.

---

1. *fen:* 1/10 of a *cun*, which is a unit of measurement equal to the inside length of the second section of the patient's own middle finger. The *cun* is measured between the ends of the creases formed when the finger is bent.

DIAGRAM 57

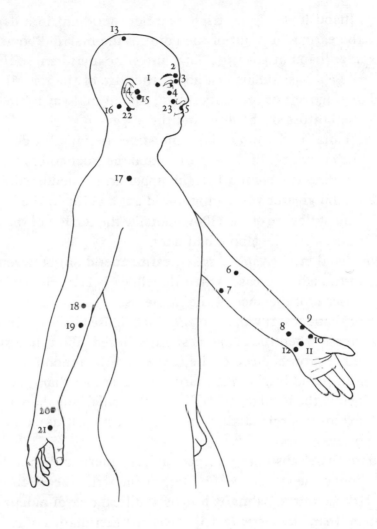

Commonly-Used Acupoints: Lateral View

1. *Taiyang*	7. *Shaohai*	13. *Baihui*	19. *Shousanli*
2. *Zuanzhu*	8. *Neiguan*	14. *Tinggong*	20. *Yangxi*
3. *Jingming*	9. *Lieque*	15. *Tinghui*	21. *Hegu*
4. *Sibai*	10. *Taiyuan*	16. *Fengchi*	22. *Yifeng*
5. *Renzhong*	11. *Daling*	17. *Jianyu*	23. *Yingxiang*
6. *Chize*	12. *Shenmen*	18. *Quchi*	

Yifeng: (hand lesser *yang*, triple warmer meridian) in a depression behind the earlobe in front of the point of the mastoid bone..

Yingxiang: (hand bright *yang*, large intestine meridian) in the depression on the ala nasi sulcus just above the edge of the nostril.

Renzhong: (governor vessel meridian) a point midway in the groove between the bottom of the nose and the upper lip.

Jianyu: (hand bright *yang*, large intestine meridian) a depression between the outer edge of the acromion and the trochanter major of the humerus. Find the point when the upper arm is abducted.

Chize: (hand greater *yang*, lung meridian) a point in the depression on the line of flexure of the elbow, outside the tendon of the biceps. Find the point with the elbow half bent.

Quchi: (hand bright *yang*, large intestine meridian) between the lateral end of the elbow crease, when the elbow is bent at a right angle, and the outer protuberance of the humerus.

Shaohai: (hand lesser *yin*, heart meridian) close to the inner end of the elbow crease when the elbow is slightly flexed: about half way between the inner protuberance of the elbow and the tendon of the biceps.

Shousanli: (hand bright *yang*, large intestine meridian) a point about 2 *cun* below the bend of the elbow on the radial side, between the musculus extensor carpi radialis longus and the musculus extensor carpi radialis brevis.

Neiguan: (hand absolute *yin*, pericardium meridian) in a depression 2 *cun* above the crease on the front of the wrist, between the two tendons (those of the palmaris longus and flexor carpi radialis muscles).

Waiguan: (hand lesser *yang*, triple warmer meridian) a point 2 *cun* above the skin crease on the back of the wrist, directly opposite *neiguan*.

Lieque: (hand greater *yang*, lung meridian) upon the anterior surface of the forearm, 1.5 *cun* above the crease of the wrist, just to the outer side of the radial artery.

Hegu: (hand bright *yang*, large intestine meridian) in the depression between the first and second metacarpal bones, near the angle formed where they meet.

Yangxi: (hand bright *yang*, large intestine meridian) in the "anatomical

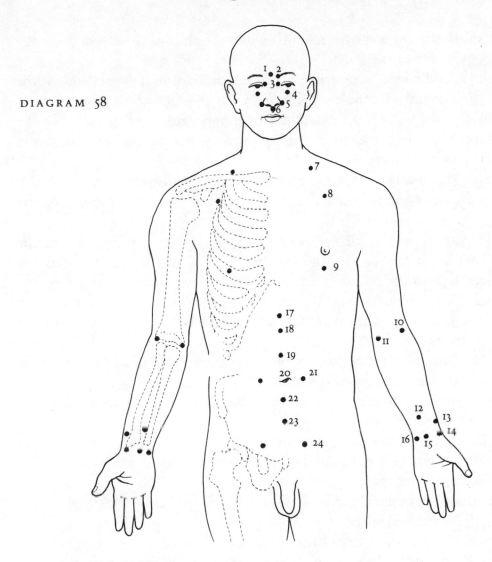

DIAGRAM 58

Commonly-Used Acupoints: Anterior View

1. *Yintang*	7. *Quepen*	13. *Lieque*	19. *Xiawan*
2. *Zuanzhu*	8. *Zhongfu*	14. *Taiyuan*	20. *Shenque*
3. *Jingming*	9. *Rugen*	15. *Daling*	21. *Tianshu*
4. *Sibai*	10. *Chize*	16. *Shenmen*	22. *Qihai*
5. *Yingxiang*	11. *Shaohai*	17. *Shangwan*	23. *Guanyuan*
6. *Renzhong*	12. *Neiguan*	18. *Zhongwan*	24. *Qichong*

snuffbox" formed by 2 tendons when the thumb is extended, on the outer side of the wrist.

Yangchi: (hand lesser *yang,* triple warmer meridian) in a depression on the back of the wrist below the base of the 4th metacarpal bone.

Yanggu: (hand greater *yang,* small intestine meridian) in a depression on the inner side of the wrist in the hollow between the tip of the ulna and the carpal bones.

Shenmen: (hand lesser *yin,* heart meridian) in a depression between the pisiform bone and the ulna on the inner (medial) side of the crease on the front of the wrist.

Daling: (hand absolute *yin,* pericardium meridian) in a depression in the middle of the crease line on the front of the wrist (between the tendons of the palmaris longus and flexor carpi radialis muscles.)

Taiyuan: (hand greater *yang,* lung meridian) in a depression on the outer side of the radial artery, at the outer end of the crease line on the front of the wrist.

Ten xuan: (irregular acupoints not on a meridian) on the tips of each of the ten fingers, 1 *fen* from the nail.

Quepen: (foot bright *yang,* stomach meridian) a depression above the clavicle, directly above the nipple.

Zhongfu: (hand greater *yang,* lung meridian) on a level with the second rib about 1 *cun* below the depression below the clavicle and medial to the coracoid process.

Rugen: (foot bright *yang,* stomach meridian) 1.6 *cun* below the nipple at the 5th intercostal space.

Shangwan: (conception vessel meridian) 5 *cun* above the navel. (The distance from the depression at the lower end of the sternum to the navel is 8 *cun*.

Zhongwan: (conception vessel meridian) 4 *cun* above the navel.

Xiawan: (conception vessel meridian) 2 *cun* above the navel.

Shenque: (conception vessel meridian) the navel itself.

Qihai: (conception vessel meridian) 1.5 *cun* below the navel. (The distance from the navel to the pubic bone is 5 *cun*.)

Guanyuan: (conception vessel meridian) 3 *cun* below the navel.

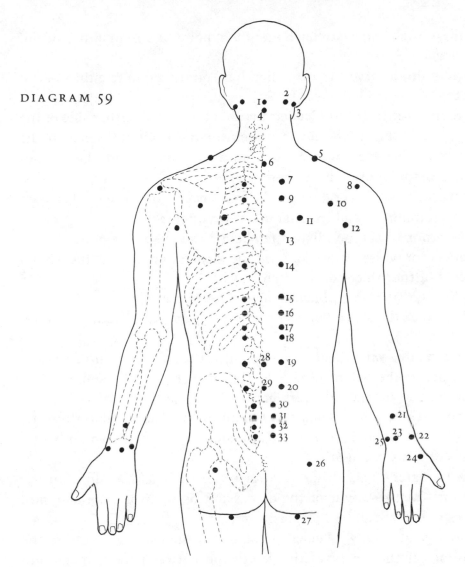

DIAGRAM 59

Commonly-Used Acupoints: Posterior View

1. *Fengfu*	9. *Feishu*	17. *Pishu*	25. *Yanggu*
2. *Fengchi*	10. *Tianzong*	18. *Weishu*	26. *Huantiao*
3. *Yifeng*	11. *Gaohuang*	19. *Shenshu*	27. *Chengfu*
4. *Yamen*	12. *Jianzhen*	20. *Dachangshu*	28. *Mingmen*
5. *Jianjing*	13. *Xinshu*	21. *Waiguan*	29. *Yangguan*
6. *Dazhui*	14. *Geshu*	22. *Yangxi*	30. *Shangliao*
7. *Fengmen*	15. *Ganshu*	23. *Yangchi*	31. *Ciliao*
8. *Jianliao*	16. *Danshu*	24. *Hegu*	32. *Zhongliao*
			33. *Xialiao*

Tianshu: (foot bright *yang*, stomach meridian) points 2 *cun* to either side of the navel.

Qichong: (foot bright *yang*, stomach meridian) points 2 *cun* to either side of the top of the pubic bone.

Fengchi: (foot lesser *yang*, gallbladder meridian) points on either side of the *fengfu* acupoint, at the lower margin of the occipital bone, in the depression between where the trapezius muscle and the sterno-cleidomastoid muscle have their origins.

Fengfu: (governor vessel meridian) in the exact center of the space between the occipital bone and the first cervical vertebra.

Yamen: (governor vessel meridian) 5 *fen* below the fengfu acupoint.

Dazhui: (governor vessel meridian) in the depression below the spinal process of the 7th cervical vertebra.

Fengmen: (foot greater *yang*, bladder meridian) bilateral points 2.0 *cun* to each side of the space between the second and third thoracic vertebrae.

Feishu: (foot greater *yang*, bladder meridian) on the back, 2 *cun* from the mid-line, at the height of the depression between the spinous processes of the 3rd and 4th vertebrae.

Xinshu: (foot greater *yang*, bladder meridian) on the back, 2 *cun* from the mid-line, at the height of the depression between the spinous processes of the 5th and 6th thoracic vertebrae.

Geshu: (foot greater *yang*, bladder meridian) on the back, 2 *cun* from the mid-line, at the height of the depression between the spinous processes of the 7th and 8th thoracic vertebrae.

Ganshu: (foot greater *yang*, bladder meridian) on the back, 2 *cun* from the mid-line, at the height of the depression between the spinous processes of the 9th and 10th thoracic vertebrae.

Danshu: (foot greater *yang*, bladder meridian) on the back, 2 *cun* from the mid-line, at the height of the depression between the spinous processes of the 10th and 11th thoracic vertebrae.

Pishu: (foot greater *yang*, bladder meridian) on the back, 2 *cun* from the mid-line, at the height of the depression between the spinous processes of the 11th and 12th thoracic vertebrae.

Weishu: (foot greater *yang*, bladder meridian) on the back, 2 *cun* from the mid-line, at the height of the depression between the spinous processes of the 12th thoracic and the first lumbar vertebrae.

Shenshu: (foot greater *yang*, bladder meridian) on the back 2 ½ *cun* from the mid-line, at the level of the depression between the 2nd and 3rd lumbar vertebrae.

Dachangshu: (foot greater *yang*, bladder meridian) 2.5 *cun* from the midline at the level of the depression between the 4th and 5th lumbar vertebrae.

Shangliao, ciliao, zhongliao, xialiao: (foot greater *yang*, bladder meridian) *Shangliao* is situated in the first posterior sacral foramen, about midway between the postero-superior iliac spine and the median line. *Ciliao* is in the second posterior sacral foramen, *zhongliao* in the third and *xialiao* in the fourth. Left and right together, there is a total of eight *liao* acupoints.

Mingmen: (governor vessel meridian) in the depression below the spinal process of the 2nd lumbar vertebra.

Yangguan: (governor vessel meridian) in the depression below the spinal process of the 4th lumbar vertebra.

Jianjing: (foot lesser *yang*, gallbladder meridian) in the depression right between the *dazhui* and *jianyu* acupoints (see above) on the front edge of the trapezius.

Jianliao: (hand lesser *yang*, triple warmer meridian) in the depression behind and below the acromion, about 1 *cun* behind the *jianyu* acupoint (see above).

Jianzhen: (hand greater *yang*, small intestine meridian) in a depression on the posterior surface of the shoulder just above the crease of the armpit.

Tianzong: (hand greater *yang*, small intestine meridian) in a depression below the mid-point of the spine of the shoulder blade.

Gaohuang: (foot greater *yang*, gallbladder meridian) on the back, 4 *cun* from the midline at the height of the depression between the spinous processes of the 4th and 5th thoracic vertebrae.

Huantiao: (foot lesser *yang*, gallbladder meridian) located on the hip behind the greater trochanter, in a depression formed in the muscle when the buttocks are tensed.

Chengfu: (foot greater *yang*, bladder meridian) on the posterior surface of each thigh, on the midpoint of the crease below the buttock.

Xuehai: (foot greater *yin*, spleen meridian) on the anterior medial surface of the thigh, 3 *cun* above the crease of the knee in the bulge of the vastus medialis muscle.

Xiyan: (irregular points not on a meridian) in the depressions on either side of the ligament below the patella; known as the inner and outer *xiyan*. Locate with the knee bent.

Zusanli: (foot bright *yang*, stomach meridian) located on the front of the leg, 3 *cun* below the patella just 1 cun lateral to the edge of the tibia.

Yanglingquan: (foot lesser *yang*, gall bladder meridian) in a depression on the side of the leg, below the head of the fibula, between the two muscles.

Juegu: foot lesser *yang*, gall bladder meridian) 3 *cun* above the lateral malleolus, between the fibula and the tibia.

Kunlun: (foot greater yang, bladder meridian) in a depression between the highest point of the lateral malleolus and the Achilles tendon.

Pucan: (foot greater *yang*, bladder meridian) 2 *cun* straight below the *kunlun* acupoint, on the outer side of the heel bone.

Yinlingquan: (foot greater *yin*, spleen meridian) in a depression below the lower margin of the medial condyle of the tibia, level with the tibial tuberosity.

Sanyinjiao: (foot greater *yang*, spleen meridian) 3 *cun* above the top of the medial malleolus, in a depression behind the tibia.

Jiexi: (foot bright *yang*, stomach meridian) located on the upper part of the instep, in the centre of the anterior crease of the ankle, between two tendons. The point is located with the knee slightly bent.

Taixi: (foot lesser *yin*, kidney meridian) in a depression between the Achilles tendon and the top of the medial malleolus, opposite *kunlun*.

Taichong: (foot absolute *yin*, liver meridian) located on the top of the foot, in the angle between the first and second metatarsal bones.

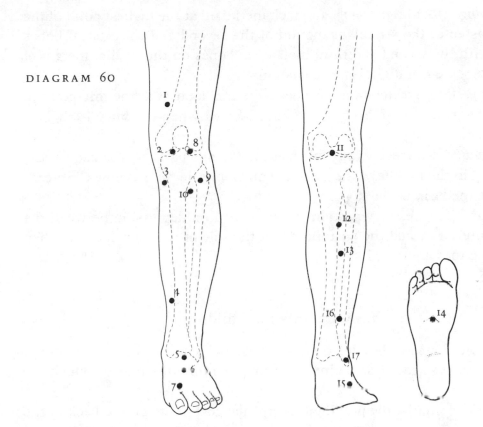

DIAGRAM 60

Commonly-Used Accupoints: Lower Limbs

1. *Xuehai*
2. *Neixiyan* (Inner *xiyan*)
3. *Yinlingquan*
4. *Sanyinjiao*
5. *Jiexi*
6. *Chongyang*
7. *Taichong*
8. *Waixiyian* (Outer *xiyan*)

9. *Yanglingquan*
10. *Zusanli*
11. *Weizhong*
12. *Chengjin*
13. *Chengshan*
14. *Yongquan*
15. *Pucan*
16. *Juegu*
17. *Kunlun*

Chongyang: (foot bright *yang*, stomach meridian) at the highest point of the instep at the articular junction of the second and third tarsal bones with the second and third metatarsal bones on the medial margin of the extensor digitorum longus muscle.

Weizhong: (foot greater *yang*, bladder meridian) a point at the mid-point of the crease at the back of the knee located when the knee is slightly bent.

Chengshan: (foot greater *yang*, bladder meridian) a point on the back of the leg in the middle of the gastrocnemius muscle 7 *cun* below the crease at the back of the knee.

Yongquan: (foot lesser *yin*, kidney meridian) in a depression between the anterior ⅓ and the posterior ⅔ of the sole of the foot, located when the toes are flexed.

2. Acupoints for Children

In pediatric massage, besides the meridians and acupoints used for adults, there are some special acupoints, the most commonly-used of which are these:

Five *zhijie:* points at the proximal interphalangeal joints on the back of the hand. The fifth is on the interphalangeal joint of the thumb.

Four *hengwen:* the four points on the palm side of the proximal interphalangeal joints.

Greater *hengwen:* at the base of the palm of the hand, on the crease of the wrist.

Lesser *hengwen:* points on the four creases where the fingers meet the palm.

Neilaogong: a point in the middle of the palm.

Two *shanmen:* in depressions on either side of the third metacarpal bone on the back of the hand.

Errenshangma: in a depression on the back of the hand between the fourth and fifth metacarpal bones.

Fanmen: in the upper part of the fleshy pad at the base of the thumb..

Yiwofeng: a point in the middle of the crease of the back of the wrist.

Waijianshi: a point on the back of the forearm, above the *waiguan* point and between the ulna and the radius.

Tianheshui: a line along the middle of the front surface of the forearm, from the wrist to the elbow crease.

Liufu: a line along the inner side of the front of the forearm from the elbow crease to the wrist.

Sanguan: a line along the outer side of the front of the forearm from the wrist to the *quchi* point at the outer end of the elbow-crease (see above).

Pitu: a line at the base of the thumb from a point on the fleshy eminence to a point on the crease of the wrist.

Dujiao: points on either side of the navel.

Guiwei: at the tip of the coccyx.

DIAGRAM 61

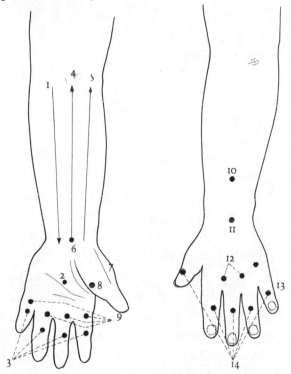

The Meridian Locations Commonly Used as Acupoints for Children

1. *Liufu*	8. *Fanmen*
2. *Neilaogong*	9. Lesser *hengwen* (*Xiaohengwen*)
3. Four *hengwen* (*Sihengwen*)	10. *Waijianshi*
4. *Tianheshui*	11. *Yiwofeng*
5. *Sanguan*	12. Two *shanmen* (*Ershanmen*)
6. Greater *hengwen* (*Dahengwen*)	13. *Errenshangma*
7. *Pitu*	14. Five *zhijie* (*Wuzhjie*)

CHAPTER IV

HOW TO USE MASSAGE THERAPY

Massage therapy is different from any other form of therapy, because the practitioner has to expend considerable physical strength in doing it, and the success of the treatment is exactly equal to the amount of effort that goes into it. This means that in the course of treatment, if you do not expend enough physical strength on a massage, you will not attain the required standard for effective treatment. On that account the therapist must work hard and not be afraid of fatigue, or of pain. You must make every effort to improve your technique. This will require much painstaking drilling. In actual clinical practice, we must continuously evaluate all our past experiences, in order to break new ground and create new methods. In this way, massage therapy will continue to be developed and brought to a still higher level.

It is necessary to tell the patient about massage therapy, to let him know that during the course of treatment some discomfort or pain may appear, and that sometimes a large number of sessions may be necessary before the treatment takes effect. Encourage patients to make up their minds not to be afraid of difficulties, and to be full of confidence that they can overcome their condition. Particularly encourage those patients with stubborn, chronic conditions to combat them with a strong will.

Section I: Actual Practice

1. Amount of Massage

It is very important that neither too much nor too little massage be given. Generally, the amount of massage will depend upon the number of massages daily, the length of time required for each massage, the intensity and the number of repetitions of each kind of manipulation, and observation of local reactions. The number of massages is determined by the requirements of different conditions. Generally, massage is applied once a day. But for some ailments, massage every other day or at a two-day interval is more appropriate. Some conditions can be treated twice a day. The duration of each massage treatment also varies. For example, where there is a sprain at a joint, localized massage and acupoint massage at the injured joint are all that is required. Generally, fifteen minutes will be quite sufficient. There are some internal diseases, however, for which massage is applied to the head, the back, the limbs, and even over the whole body. Normally, this will take thirty minutes or so. This describes the general situation, but treatment must be based upon the individual case.

In children's massage, the number of times each massage is repeated during one session is generally determined by what is required for each site. Different regions of China have developed different approaches. In some provinces, massage is applied several tens of times, in others several hundred times, and in still others even as many as 2–3,000 times. Usually, we ourselves massage a site 2–300 times, which takes about 15–25 minutes in all. For children, the amount of massage is also determined by the amount of reddening of the skin. This is a criterion that is relatively easy to weigh. For adult massage, in the case of some techniques, the amount of time required is also determined by the number of repetitions. (See details given in the treatment sections for each disease.)

2. The Degree of Force to Use in Massage

The degree of force used in massage is directly related to the amount of massage. Whether the degree of force is adequate will greatly affect the result of the treatment.

a) Proper sequence and gradual progress: Both in each massage session and in the whole course of treatment, the massage must be light at the beginning, becoming gradually heavier. The amount of force should be increased, but not so abruptly as to be unbearable to the patient.

b) When the dig method is applied at an acupoint: The dig method should reach down to a point where the vital energy (*qi*) appears, producing an aching, swelling reaction like a pin-prick, or sometimes a shooting, painful, numb sensation. The strength of these sensations is determined by the intensity of the finger-digs, and this intensity must be under skillful control. The vibrate and kneading methods can be used in coordination with the dig method in order to intensify or lessen these sensations.

c) During massage on the head and back: Here no pain should be allowed to occur, nor should the skin be damaged. Rather, the massage should give the patient a sensation of warmth, and make him or her feel relaxed and comfortable.

d) When massage therapy is applied to a wounded patient: In this case the pain in the area of the wound should be added to as little as possible. When various kinds of passive manipulation are used, the range of the passive movement, and the amount of force to be used in stretching a limb should be fully estimated at the outset, and the amount of force gradually increased to the maximum possible.

e) The strength of the manipulation: This will have a definite relation with the amount of time for which it is applied. When great force is used, a massage should be applied somewhat fewer times in a session; when little force is used, the massage should be applied somewhat more times.

3. Treat Each Case Individually

Every patient has his own individual characteristics. There are the obvious differences of sex, age, and physical constitution. But there are also marked differences between different diseases and different phases of the same disease. Hence, in applying the various massage therapy manipulations, amount of force and length of time are adjusted to the individual patient.

Some patients are relatively sensitive, and even though only a light manipulation is used, the patient feels a strong reaction. In such a case both the amount of massage and the degree of force used should be reduced. Conversely, there is often little reaction in the patient with a strong constitution, and the degree of force used should be increased. In summary, each case must be dealt with individually. Especially with a new patient, the amount of massage and degree of force used must first be tested out, and the patient's reactions observed. Then, gradually, a suitable procedure can be established.

4. Important Considerations

a) Receive the patient warmly and diagnose his/her condition in detail.

b) Before beginning, place the patient in a suitable position, such as sitting, lying, or with the affected limb raised, in order to relax the muscles and to facilitate massage.

c) The therapist should always be aware of his own position, so that it will help produce the correct force, and will also save his own energy. In general, the therapist can stand beside, behind, or facing the patient. A sitting position generally involves sitting face to face. In the standing position, the archer's and the rider's positions are both sometimes used.

d) While he is applying the massage the practitioner has to devote his entire attention to it, comfortably adjusting his breathing and carrying out the treatment whole-heartedly. In this manner, the goal of the treatment can be reached, and injury can be avoided.

e) The hands of the therapist should be kept warm and clean, and the fingernails must be trimmed often.

f) In massage sessions where no exhaustive diagnosis is to be made prior to treatment, any circumstance that may contraindicate massage must still be noted. The progress of the disease must also be discerned, the patient's reactions noted and an explanation given.

g) When massaging, be sure to proceed from site to site in the proper sequence, going from the distant points toward the center of the body. Make skillful use of the various techniques, applying them with appropriate degrees of force and in appropriate amounts.

h) If the patient is very full or very hungry, it is inadvisable to carry out the massage. Generally, it is best not to proceed with massage during the period from ½ hour before to 1½ hours after a meal.

Section II: Media Used in Massage

During massage, the therapist often puts some liquid or powder on his or her hand to reduce friction and increase lubrication, or to gain the additional benefit of a medication. These liquids or powders are called the "media" for use in massage. There are numerous kinds of media, including liquids, tinctures, oils, and powders. The most common media are these:

1) *Fresh ginger juice:* Pound fresh ginger into a mud-like consistency and put it in a container. Dip the fingers into the juice exuded by the ginger, using it as a medium for massage. This is one of the most frequently used media, and is almost always used in massage of children. Because children have soft, tender skin and because the ginger juice is very slippery, the skin is unlikely to be abraded during massage. At the same time, the ginger juice produces a radiating warmth and helps to dispel harmful external influences.[1]

2) *Cold water:* If ginger juice is not available, substitute clean, cold tap-water. Especially when a child has a fever, cold water is often used as a medium.

3) *Shavings water:* Soak wood shavings in water, and use the resulting liquid as a medium. Shavings water is very slippery and is therefore also very suitable for massage of children.

4) *Egg white:* Make a small hole in an egg shell, extract the egg white from the shell, and use it as a medium. The egg white can also be mixed with flour to make a dough-ball. The practitioner holds the dough-ball in his hand and applies the rub-roll, the rub, and the roll methods on a child's chest, abdomen, and back areas. This medium is often used in the folk treatment of children's influenza, "food build-up"[2] and other illnesses.

---

1. This refers to a concept of Chinese medicine whereby diseases can be caused by certain external factors, the most important of which are heat, cold, wind, moisture, and warmth.
2. Food build-up: a condition described by Chinese medicine in which the patient eats too much and undigested food builds up inside of him.

5) *Songhua powder:* Pulverize Songhua into a fine powder. Use this powder as a medium by dipping the fingers into it or by applying it directly with a powder-puff to the site to be massaged. It acts to absorb moisture and increase lubrication. In summer, when the skin perspires easily, use of this powder is especially appropriate.

6) *Talcum powder:* Generally, talcum powder used medically is chiefly for its lubricating effect.

7) *Strong liquor*[3]*:* This is used mainly on adults. It acts to invigorate the blood and to dispel the ills resulting from wind, cold, and moisture. It can also lower the temperature of a patient with fever.

8) *Medicinal liquor for external use:* Soak various Chinese medicinal herbs in strong liquor. After a few days, you can use the resulting liquid as a medium. The generally-used Chinese medicinal herbs all belong to the group of drugs used for moving the vital energy and invigorating the blood. Several frequently-used prescriptions follow.[4] (See Appendix for Table of Weights.)

(i)

Ruxiang	Boswellia glabra (frankincense)	1 *qian*
Moyao	Commiphora myrrha Engler (myrrh)	1 *qian*
Shenshanqi	Rhus verniciflua Stokes	1 *qian*
Tibetan *honghua*	Carthamus tinctorius (safflower)	1 *qian*
(Szechuan *honghua* may be used instead)		
Meibingpian	Dryobalanops camphora Coleb. (borneol)	2 *fen*
Guangmuxiang	Saussurea lappa Clarke (costusroot)	3 *fen*
Zhangnao	Camphor	2 *qian*
Xuejie	Daemonorops draco Blume (dragon's blood)	3 *qian*

The above herbs are soaked in two catties of strong liquor for a period of two weeks. The mixture is appropriate for acute and chronic injuries.

---

3. Strong liquor: refers to *gaoliang*, brandy, whisky, grade A rice wine, etc. Chinese liquors are usually 65% alcholol.
4. Chinese medicinal herbs are available in cities with large Chinese populations, in herbal medicine shops, and some Chinese grocery stores.

(ii) *Honghua*   Carthamus tinctorius L. (safflower)

    Chuanwu   Aconitum carmichaeli Debx. (prepared root)

    Caowu   Aconitum chinense Pext. (root)

    Guiwei   Angelica sinensis (root ends)

    Taoren   Prunus persica (peach kernel)

    Gancao (fresh)   Licorice-root

    Jiang (fresh)   Ginger-root

    Mahuang   Ephedra vulgaris

    Duanzirantong   Native copper

    Maqianzi   Strychnos nux vomica L. (nut)

    Guizhi   Cinnamomum cassia Blume (sticks)

    Ruxiang   Boswellia glabra (frankincense)

    Moyao   Commiphora myrrha Engler (myrrh)

Soak 1 *liang* of each of the above thirteen herbs in 3 catties of strong liquor for two weeks. The mixture is suitable for general injuries, and is especially effective in the treatment of acute and chronic injuries of bone or cartilage.

(iii) *Mahuang* (fresh)	Ephedra vulgaris	7 *qian*
Sangzhi	Morus alba L. (mulberry twigs)	3 *qian*
Fangfeng	Saposhnikovia divaricata (root)	2 *qian*
Wushaoshe	Zaocys dhumnades (snake)	4 *qian*
Tianchong	Dried silkworm	1 *qian*
Honghua	Carthamus tinctorius L. (safflower)	5 *qian*
Chuanwu (fresh)	Aconitum carmichaeli Debx. (root)	3 *qian*
Baizhi	Angelica anomala (root)	2 *qian*
Qianghuo	Notopterygium incisum Ting. (root)	1 *qian*
Duhuo	Angelica pubescens Maxim. (root)	1 *qian*
Baixianpi	Dictamnus dasycarpus (root bark)	2 *qian*
Xixiancao	Siegesbeckia orientalis var. pubescens (leaves)	3 *qian*

The above twelve kinds of herb soaked in three catties of *Gaoliang* (sorghum) liquor for two weeks are suitable for poliomyelitis, and child pneumonia.

(iv) Fresh green onion and ginger in equal amounts, soaked in 95% alcohol for two weeks is suitable for children with the common cold.

9) *Yushushenyou* (cajuputi oleum): This is a synthesized Chinese medicine that acts as a resolvent and an analgesic. It is often used as a medium in massage of wounds.

10) *Sesame oil:* This has the chief effect of increasing lubrication. It is often used as a medium in the "scraping" and "twist" methods of Chinese folk medicine.

11) *Chuandaoyou* ("conduction oil"): This is a medium first used in Shanghai. It is composed of cajuputi oil (see 9 above), glycerin, turpentine, alcohol, and distilled water. It can reduce swelling, kill pain, and dispel the effects of wind and cold.

12) *Cinnamon oil:* Cinnamon is fragrant and promotes warmth. It is used as a medium in deficiency ailments caused by cold.

13) *Zhanjindan*[5] "Muscle-stretching powder," also called "kneading medication." Grind the following seven herbs into a fine powder and pack in a sealed bottle for later use. *Zhanjindan* acts as a resolvent and an analgesic and is mostly used as a medium for massage when there has been an injury.

Ruxiang	Boswellia glabra (frankincense)	2 *qian*
Moyao	Commiphora myrrha Engler (myrrh)	2 *qian*
Tibetan *honghua*	Carthamus tinctorius L. (safflower)	1 *qian*
Shexiang	Musk	5 *fen*
Bingpian	Dryobalanops camphora (borneol)	5 *fen*
Zhangnao	Camphor	5 *fen*
Xuejie	Daemonorops draco Blume (dragon's blood)	5 *qian*

---

5. *"Dan"* has many different meanings. Here it refers to a pulvis of dried herbs, triturated and mixed in the amounts specified. The word can also refer to a pill, troche or magna, to cinnabar, to alchemy or to a panacea.

Section III: Massage Therapy
in Conjunction with Other Treatments

Clinically, a choice is made according to the nature of the illness as to which of various methods of treatment is to be primary and which secondary. Massage therapy is often the primary method of treatment for certain conditions, such as protrusion of a lumbar intervertebral disk or rheumatoid spondylitis. In some other ailments, such as bedsores, massage therapy is used as an accessory measure, in coordination with other methods of treatment.

Several treatment methods are frequently recommended for use in conjunction with massage therapy:

1. Massage therapy and Medical Exercise (Taoist Yoga)

Medical exercise is a form of therapeutic gymnastic training. In China in ancient times it was called "Taoist yoga," and was often associated with massage. It can be seen that massage and Taoist yoga were already known in ancient times to be closely related. Both massage and yogic exercises are used in treating certain diseases. While the former is a passive method, the latter is a method involving active movement. These two methods, when combined, can give the patient a better recovery. Therefore, during the course of massage it is also important to instruct the patient in medical exercise. From the long-range point of view, the medical exercise is more important than the massage, because it can fully develop the patient's capacities to positively combat his illness. It can have a marked effect on victory over disease, consolidation of therapeutic effect, and recovery and development of ability to work. (For details of methods of medical exercise see the sections on the treatment of specific conditions.)

2. Chinese Herbal Fomentations

At the end of each massage session in cases of injury or rheumatic illness, a warm, wet compress of Chinese herbs is often used to heighten the effect of the treatment. Prescriptions reflect the requirements of different diseases.

Generally, drugs are used that help realign the tissues and activate blood circulation.

Directions for herbal compresses: Pack the herbs in a gauze bag, place them in a pot, add clean water. Then add two thicknesses of towelling (or six to eight layers of gauze or linen sewn together into a rectangular cushion) and immerse them in the water. The amount of water should be sufficient to soak through the cloth. As soon as it comes to a boil, take out one towel. Wring it dry, fold to size and, while it is still hot, spread it over the affected area. Take care that it is not too hot, so as to avoid scalding the skin. After a 1–2 minute interval take out the other towel, wring it dry and change towels. Continue doing this ten or more times in succession. Afterwards see that the skin is rubbed dry and the affected area kept warm, and make sure that the patient is not subjected to drafts or cold. Where conditions permit, 4–6 layers of towel can be spread over the affected area, the outside wrapped with oilcloth and covered with a cotton blanket. In this way the heat will not dissipate so easily. This will permit changing towels at 7–10 minute intervals, and will make 2–3 changes sufficient.

Note: Prescription for a fomentation of Chinese medicinal herbs:

Qianghuo	Notopterygium incisum Ting. (root)
Duhuo	Angelica pubescens Maxim. (root)
Ruxiang (fresh)	Boswellia glabra (frankincense)
Moyao (fresh)	Commiphora myrrha Engler (myrrh)
Chuanwu (fresh)	Aconitum carmichaeli Debx. (root)
Caowu (fresh)	Aconitum chinense Pext. (root)
Shenjincao	Lycopodium cernuum L.
Guizhi	Cinnamomum cassia Blume (sticks)
Mugua	Chaenomeles lagenaria Koidz.(fruit)
Lulutong	Liquidambar formosana
Shichangpu	Acorus gramineus Soland. (root)
Dibiechong	Larrada aurulenta (beetle)
Honghua	Carthamus tinctorius L. (safflower)

Use 3 *qian* of each of the above 13 ingredients.

3. Massage in Setting Fractures

This is a treatment method which closely combines reduction of fractures with massage. First, manipulation is used to bring the fracture to a correct position. Then, during the entire course of treatment, frequent massage and realignment are carried out. This static/dynamic approach is the main feature of traditional Chinese medical thought on the management of fractures. (For further discussion see the section "Fractures of the Limbs," p. 133.)

4. Other Treatments

Physical therapy, acupuncture, hypodermically administered herbal medications, etc., are often applied in conjunction with massage therapy.

Section IV: Applications of and Contraindications to Massage Therapy

1. Applications

There is extensive scope for the application of massage therapy. It can be used for numerous diseases in the fields of internal, surgical, pediatric, and traumatic medicine. Generally speaking, massage therapy is suitable for chronic and functional diseases. However, it can also have a good therapeutic effect in certain acute illnesses, such as the common cold, acute sprains, etc. The traumatic conditions it is most used in include acute sprain, contusion, chronic strain, a lumbar slipped intervertebral disk, and fractures of the limbs. The internal diseases it is most used in are the common cold, acute gastroenteritis, ulcers, gastroptosis, paralysis, and rheumatoid arthritis. The pediatric diseases where massage therapy is most frequently used are acute upper respiratory tract infections, digestive disturbances, chronic nutritional disturbances, and poliomyelitis.

2. Contraindications

Although there is extensive scope for application of massage therapy, there are also definite contraindications to its use. Based on the understanding gained in our practice, here are some points regarding the areas of contraindication.

1) Acute infectious diseases such as diphtheria, typhoid fever, etc.

2) Various kinds of skin diseases. If the areas of the skin disease are excluded, massage can still be carried out on the healthy areas.

3) Various types of tumor, particularly the area of a malignant tumor.

4) Psychosis.

5) When abscesses and pyemia are present.

6) The intensifying stages of pulmonary tuberculosis, vertebral tuberculosis and multiple tuberculosis, etc.

7) If a hemorrhagic disorder may occur when massage is administered.

8) For a patient in a critical condition.

9) Massage therapy is generally contraindicated for pregnant women.

10) Massage is inadvisable when the patient is extremely fatigued, or intoxicated.

CHAPTER V

CLINICAL APPLICATIONS
OF MASSAGE THERAPY

1. Protrusion of a Lumbar
Intervertebral Disk (Slipped Disk)

Protrusion of a lumbar intervertebral disk is also known as rupture of a lumbar intervertebral fibrous ring. It is usually due to injury which causes the tissue of the nucleus pulposus of the intervertebral disk between two vertebral bodies to bulge out or become dislocated. This gives rise to lumbar pain on one side of the body and in the leg. The condition is common among working people. Massage therapy is uniquely effective in treating it.

Etiology and Pathology

There is usually a history of obvious injury, such as suddenly wrenching the lower back while lifting or carrying a heavy load. There is great elasticity and tenacity in the human spinal column, which acts to buffer any outside force. However, when the outside force is too great, going beyond what the fibrous ring around the circumference of the intervertebral disk can absorb, then the fibrous ring will crack and the structure of the nucleus pulposus will bulge out or be dislocated, leading to this condition. On the other hand, in some cases there is no obvious traumatic history, retrogressive changes having previously developed in the tissue of the intervertebral disk due to weak structure, spinal disease, or old age. Under these conditions, only a slight outside force, or even a sudden uncoordinated muscle contraction can result in this condition. For example, we have had a case in which the condition was attributed to the lumbar region's having been attacked by cold.

Symptoms

The main symptoms of this condition are usually low back pain, pain radiating down the lower extremities, disturbance of sensation in the lower limbs, difficulty in walking, and postural changes.

a) Low back pain: This complaint seldom occurs without low back pain. Often, at its onset, there is a stab of severe pain in the lumbar region, so intense that any movement of the lower back dare not be attempted. In the course of the pathogenic process the pain that has developed in the lower back area will gradually get better, but the pain in the leg area will be aggravated. The pain of the lumbar region often tends to be on one side. Sitting or walking will tend to aggravate it, while bed rest will alleviate it.

b) Pain radiating to the lower extremities: Pain is radiated to the lower limb on the same side. This is caused by the protruded intervertebral disk pushing against the related nerve roots in the spinal canal. Most often this occurs in the 4th or 5th lumbar intervertebral disk. The pain may radiate along the course of the sciatic nerve down the back of the knee, the lateral side of the calf, or the sole of the foot, mostly reaching the calf area. In a few cases, the 3rd lumbar intervertebral disk is pushed out, and the radial pain in the lower limb will radiate along the femoral nerve from the antero-lateral aspect of the thigh down to the knee area. The pain will be persistent and convulsive. At the onset of the disease the pain is unbearable, and the patient cannot either sit or lie in comfort. Only if the body is placed in a better position, can the pain be somewhat reduced. Whenever the thigh is raised, the waist bent, or the patient sneezes or coughs, the disorder will be aggravated.

c) Disturbance of sensation in the lower limbs: This will vary according to the site and degree of the protrusion. When the protruded part is in the 4th lumbar intervertebral space, a decrease in skin sensation, will occur on the outside of the patient's calf. When the bulged part is in the 5th lumbar intervertebral space, the sole of the patient's foot, especially the big toe, will develop a decrease in skin sensation. In addition, the patient may have a feeling of numbness and numb-like pain in the affected limb, the temperature of the limb on the affected side will feel abnormal, and the amount of perspiration on the two lower limbs will not be the same.

d) *Difficulty in walking and postural change:* Different degrees of difficulty in walking will be produced according to the position of the protrusion, the connections of the pinched nerve roots and the condition's stage of development. In general, the patient will not dare to support himself because of the pain in the affected limb, and at the same time because he does not take a full stride, varying degrees of limp will be seen. Serious cases will not be able to get up from bed, and will keep the affected leg bent, not daring to stretch it out and lie flat. It becomes extremely inconvenient to have to turn over on the bed.

The affected person will generally also show postural change. Frequently the lumbar spine will curve out toward the affected side, in a few cases towards the healthy side. The buttocks of the affected side will stick out backwards and the upper part of the body will slant somewhat forward.

Diagnosis

A preliminary diagnosis can be made on the basis of history and symptoms. But this must still be confirmed by the following examination:

a) *Tender pressure point in the paravertebral muscles:* On the side of the intervertebral space to which the disk is protruding, not far from the midline of the spinal column, there is generally a fixed tender point. Its location can be determined by repeated pressing; this will help to establish the location of the protrusion. While there is a local pressure pain in this area, it also usually radiates down to the buttocks and the lower limb on the same side. The presence of a pressure pain is generally easily determined, though sometimes it is necessary to press deeply with the thumb in order to find it. In a minority of cases there is no obvious fixed point of tenderness in the paravertebral muscles, but only a sensitive area. When that area is hammered with the fist, pain will radiate into the lower limb on the same side.

b) *Straight-leg elevation test:* The patient lies on his or her back, with both legs extended. When the affected leg is elevated about 40° or less from the bed, a pulling radiating pain is immediately felt in the lumbar region and in the postero-lateral part of the thigh. This means that the straight-leg elevation test is positive. The pain is the result of tension in the compressed nerve roots. Thus, the degree to which this test is positive will depend upon how much the nerve roots are being pressed by the protruded part, and the degree of the inflammation in the compressed nerve roots. In mild cases the straightened leg can be elevated higher, while in severe cases there will immediately be pain when the leg is only slightly lifted from the surface of the bed. Some patients cannot even stretch out the affected leg. In still other cases, elevation of the sound leg can cause pain on the affected side in the lumbar area in the leg. This is called "cross-pain." The presence of this phenomenon is extremely helpful in diagnosing this condition.

c) *Neck-bending test:* Here the patient lies on his back with both legs extended. The doctor uses his hands to support the patient's head, first bending the neck slightly forward, then suddenly bending it forward with some force. If the patient complains of pain in the lower back and leg on the affected side, the neck-bending test can be considered positive. The cause of the pain is the upper part of the nerve roots being pressed by the protruded area. When the neck is bent the spinal cord is pulled upward, resulting in a painful reaction in the pressed nerve roots. This examination is also very helpful in diagnosis.

d) *Knee and Achilles tendon reflex tests:* Abnormalities often appear in the reflexes of the knee or Achilles tendon on the affected side, depending on the site of the protrusion. In cases of protrusion of the 4th or 5th lumbar intervertebral disk, weakening or disappearance of the Achilles tendon reflex usually occurs. In a few cases, the reflex becomes hyperactive.

e) *The bending back of the big toe test:* Here the patient lies on his back with both legs extended straight, bending the big toe backwards. The therapist presses the big toes down in the opposite direction judging whether there is any difference in the amount of force with which the two big toes are bent backwards. The nerve roots pressed by the protruded area often bring about a decrease in the strength of the extensor muscles of the lower limb, especially of the calf. Hence, the big toe on the affected side is always either weaker than that on the healthy side or even totally unable to bend backward. This phenomenon is often most apparent where it is the 5th lumbar intervertebral disk that is protruded. In general, such a decrease of muscular strength will appear as soon as this condition sets in.

f) Muscular atrophy: Often this condition produces muscular atrophy in the thigh and leg. Frequently this is clearly visible in the muscle group at the front of the shin and it generally manifests itself in cases where the condition has a comparatively long course. Palpation is used to determine the size and tension of the belly of the muscle. The degree of muscle atrophy can also be determined by measuring the circumference of the leg.

g) X-ray examination: An x-ray is made of the lumbo-sacral spine, so that other pathological changes in the bones of the lumbar spine and the sacro-iliac area can be eliminated from consideration. By this method we can also find secondary results of the protrusion of a disk, such as lateral curvature of the vertebral column, disappearance of the physiological arch of lordosis, narrowing of the intervertebral space, and various pathological changes in the posterior facet joint articulations. However, all these phenomena usually occur only after the course of the disease has become prolonged, and x-ray examination can therefore only be used as an auxiliary diagnosis.

Treatment

First, the diagnosis must be correct, the phase of the disease clearly distinguished, and limitations in lumbar mobility, etc. determined. Based on all these factors satisfactory therapeutic effect can be reached through choice based on all of the proper therapeutic techniques.

a) Massage: Based on our own practical experience, we feel that in deciding which massage techniques to employ, the following general treatment situations should be distinguished:

I. *Light manipulation:* In mild cases the light application of massage is judged to produce good results. In very severe cases, since heavy massage would cause great pain, light massage can be used at first. The sequence of this sort of manipulation is as follows:

(i) *Preparation:* First the patient lies face down. The chest and abdominal areas are each supported with a pillow. In very severe cases where the patient cannot lie face down, more pillows can be placed beneath the chest and abdomen. The patient put his hands by the side of his body, and relaxes his muscles.

(ii) *Muscle relaxation:* With the thumb or the base of the palm of one or both hands, the practitioner kneads with a circular motion up and down along either side of the lumbar spine and the buttocks, going from top to bottom and then bottom to top. Force is gradually increased and the process is repeated 3–4 times. At intervals the thumb push and thumb kneading methods can be applied to acupoints such as *mingmen*, *shenshu*, eight *liao*, *huantiao*, *weizhong*, and *chengshan*. Finally, the roll method is applied, going downward along the lumbar region and leg of the affected side. With these methods it will take about 10 minutes to relax the muscles.

(iii) *Stretching:* Tell the patient to turn onto his side, with the affected side upward. The practitioner stands behind the patient and applies the lumbar stretch method, Type 1. (See Diagram 44, page 46.) The patient actively relaxes his muscles and the therapist forcefully bends the hip and knee joints forward. He gradually increases the amount to which the hip-joint bends, carrying it forward with a rhythmic and elastic movement. This is done in such a way that the patient does not experience severe pain. As the degree of bending of the hip is increased, the lower lumbar vertebrae will undergo the effects of the bending force. Then, each time the hip has been bent forward 4–5 times, the hand supporting the affected leg pulls the leg out backwards with a strong and dexterous shaking motion. Meanwhile the other hand, which is against the lumbar region, presses forward with an appropriate amount of force. The rhythm of this pressing must be coordinated with that of the backward extension of the leg. The degree of force should be accommodated to what the patient can tolerate. Therefore, when stretching the patient's back, carefully take note of its potential mobility and watch the patient's facial expression. The movement must be performed rhythmically, dexterously and with force, but violence must be avoided. The entire procedure may be repeated 2–3 times.

(iv) *Moving the leg (the lower-limb stretch):* Next ask the patient to turn over onto his back for "moving the leg," the lower-limb stretch method. (See

Diagram 49, page 50.) For this, ask the patient to follow the force exerted by the therapist, and to relax the muscles as much as possible. The angle formed between the leg and the surface of the bed will at first be less than the angle reached at the time of the straight-leg elevation test. But during the procedure, carefully observe how far the affected leg can be raised, and gradually raise it higher and higher. Sometimes both legs will need "moving." Do each side about 20 times.

b) *Strong backward extension:* This is appropriate where the patient has been in the chronic phase of the disease for several months or years; where the painful symptoms have already improved; where, though the pain is still quite severe, the patient's strong constitution allows him/her to put up with a much heavier manipulation; where the patient's lumbar area is soft and flexible; where all the techniques described earlier have been used without producing any obvious results; or where the patient with severe symptoms has had his pain take a turn for the better after the application of the aforementioned massage techniques. Strong backward extension of the lumbar area is suitable under all these conditions.

(i) The patient lies face down. Apply the kneading and roll methods to the lumbar and leg areas, causing the muscles to relax, as described before.

(ii) The lumbar stretch method, type 3, is performed. (See Diagram 46, page 47.) Sometimes, when doing the strong backward extension, a crack may be heard in the patient's lumbar area. When this occurs, a better result is likely.

(iii) Perform the lumbar stretch method, type 4. (See Diagram 47, page 48.) In this action, the pulling of the leg must be coordinated with the foot pushing against the lumbar region. With this sudden movement a cracking sound may sometimes be heard in the joints of the lumbar region. Where this occurs a better effect will probably result. After this manipulation, the patient is placed face down, and massage is applied on the lower back by means of the kneading and roll methods.

(iv) Next, the patient lies on his back, and the lower-limb stretch is performed as previously described.

(v) In some cases the slanting backward extension method may be added. Here, the patient lies face down. The therapist stands on the patient's un-

Application of the techniques

(i) In performing the lumbar stretch method, it is first necessary to note whether pain is caused by bending the lumbar area forward, or by extending it backward. In severe cases, pain is generally caused by extending it backward. In performing the manipulation, the forward bending should be done first. The strength and extent of this forward bending must be great enough to produce an effect upon the spinal column. Gradually, with a shaking motion, pull the affected leg out straight. Then, by degrees, pull it out backward. Finally, apply force to the spine, making the vertebral column stretch backward elastically. In a few cases, bending the lumbar area forward is painful. In such cases, the backward extension of the hips should be done first, and the forward bending after it. The extent and the strength of the manipulations should be as above.

(ii) After several treatments, when the therapist finds that the backward extending action has helped the patient, then the extent and strength of the backward extension should gradually be increased. At the same time, the leg can be "moved" backward. In this method the patient lies face downward while the therapist uses one hand to apply the roll method to the patient's lumbar region on the afflicted side; with the other arm he holds the kneecap and leg of the same side. While the one hand presses down as it rolls, the other hand moves the leg backwards. The rhythm of this operation must be coordinated between the two hands. The extent to which the leg is moved backward should be gradually increased.

(iii) After several treatments, when the therapist finds that the forward bending motion has helped the patient, the extent and strength of the forward bending should gradually be increased. Meanwhile the two-hip bend method can be applied. (See Diagram 37, page 40.)

(iv) *Try always to act as early as possible in the course of a disease!* With cases in their early stages, the extent and strength of the movements should be increased as soon as possible. In some cases the lumbar twist method can be added: the patient lies on his side, with the afflicted side up. The lumbar area is cushioned with a thick pillow. Standing behind the patient, the practitioner holds the patient's shoulder area with one hand, and the other holds the crest of the ilium. Then he twists the lumbar area back and forth 4–5 times.

affected side and graps the ankle of the affected side with one hand, holding down the lumbo-sacral area with the other hand. The affected leg is forcibly drawn backward and toward the therapist. The other essentials of this technique are as in (iii) above.

c) *Treading:* This method may be applied in cases where the condition has already lasted for a long time, months or years; where the patient is heavily built, or his lumbar area is comparatively solid and strong; where the methods described above do not achieve a satisfactory degree of bending of the lumbar spine; or where, after the previous methods have been tried, though there is some improvement, the patient's condition remains unsatisfactory. In all these circumstances, the tread method is suitable. (See Diagram 50, page 51.)

Before applying the tread method, it is important to first clear away the patient's apprehensions about this method, and to bring about a situation where therapist and patient can work in cooperation. Tell the patient to follow the rise and fall of the treading movement with his breathing, and to breathe with his/her mouth wide open. The strength of the treading should, according to the degree of mobility of the patient's lumbar spine be gradually increased, up to what the patient is able to stand. One bout of treading, going from light to heavy, generally requires about 20–50 steps. For the last several steps in the bout of treading, the intensity should be as great as the patient is able to bear. While applying the tread method, the practitioner carefully observes the intensity the patient can endure, gradually proceeding from light to heavy, and doing so rhythmically, gently, and firmly. No violent movement is to be made at any time. Each treatment will include from two to three bouts, and during each treatment try to reach as sufficient a degree of force as possible. Between each bout, take several minutes rest. The tread method should not be carried out every day. There should be 1–2 days of rest before this treatment is resumed.

At the end of an application of the tread method, the patient is told to turn over onto his back. Then the lower-limb stretch method is repeated, as described above.

If the tread method alone were applied to some patients where it is the fifth lumbar, intervertebral disk that is protruded, there would not be a positive therapeutic effect. If traction is first applied, and is then accompanied by the

tread method, there will be a much better effect. This requires the help of two assistants: one pulls the patient by the armpits, using his hands or a broad belt; the other pulls the patient's legs in the opposite direction. Then the tread method is applied.

d) Other Treatments: In addition to massage, where conditions allow, physical therapy, Chinese herbal fomentations, and medicated poultices may be used. Medical exercise is very useful in heightening and consolidating therapeutic effect and preventing relapse. Taking the patient's condition into account, these should be applied as soon as possible. Before applying the tread method, an anodyne can be orally or hypodermically administered to some more sensitive patients.

(i) *Chinese herbal prescription for medicated poultices:* The following ten Chinese herbs are all crushed into a powder, decocted with vinegar and mixed into a paste, then applied externally on the painful part of the lumbar area, while still hot:

Caowu (fresh)	Aconitum chinense Pext. (root)
Ruxiang (fresh)	Boswellia glabra (frankincense)
Moyao (fresh)	Commiphora myrrha Engler (myrrh)
Xuejie	Daemonorops draco Blume (dragon's blood)
Jixingzi	Impatiens balsamiha L. (seeds)
Dibiechong	Larrada aurulenta (beetle)
Shangrougui	Cinnamomum cassia Blume
Qianghuo	Notopterygium incisum Ting. (root)
Duhuo	Angelica pubescens Maxim. (root)
Chuanwu (fresh)	Aconitum carmichaeli Debx. (root)

The quantity for each of the above ten herbs is 1 *liang*.

Therapeutic Effect

The diagnosis must be accurate in order to cure this condition by massage, and the correct manipulations must be selected according to various phases and conditions of the condition. The success rate is quite high. In some acute

Medical exercise

a) Moving the hips: The patient lies on his back. First, he vigorously extends his right leg, simultaneously swinging his hips to the right. (See Diagram 62.) Then he does the same with his left leg. The movements should be well-coordinated and energetic. Alternate legs 20–30 times.

b) Leg-kick: The patient lies on his back. He bends his hip and knee joints as far as possible, with the instep bent backward as well. Then he kicks his heel upward forcefully at a 45° angle. After kicking out, keep the muscles of the thigh and leg tense. (See Diagram 63.) Then lower the leg to its original position. Alternate legs 20–60 times.

DIAGRAM 62

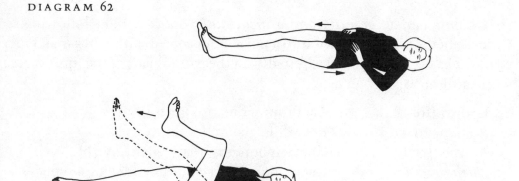

DIAGRAM 63

c) Chest-lift: Face down on the bed, the patient supports himself on his hands. Starting from the head area, he gradually raises his chest up backward until the force of the lifting reaches his waist. (See Diagram 64.) He repeats this movement 5–10 times, resting between repetitions.

d) Fish-jump: The patient lies face down, with both hands behind his back. He raises his legs and upper body at the same time, stretching

cases, where the patient has been ill for just a few days, several treatments only are needed before health is restored. In cases of somewhat longer standing, the time required for treatment is also longer. First, the patient will usually experience a relieved sensation in the leg area. Then his straight-leg elevation test will gradually improve. In some cases the buttocks may re-

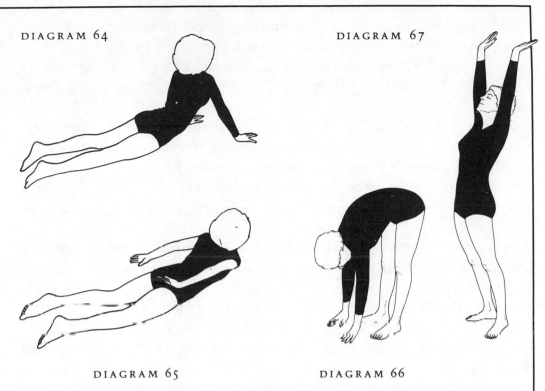

DIAGRAM 64

DIAGRAM 67

DIAGRAM 65

DIAGRAM 66

them backward so that he assumes a bowed position. He must be certain not to bend his knees. (See Diagram 65.) This posture is held as well as possible for as long as possible.

e) *Bending from the waist and backward extension:* The patient stands with feet shoulder-width apart and turned inwards. He bends forward at the waist, bouncing down until his hands touch the ground. (See Diagram 66.) Then he returns to his upright position and stretches backward at the waist, bouncing back as far as he can. (See Diagram 67.) Repeat 5–10 times. The range of the movements should increase as the patient's condition improves, but he must be sure to proceed gradually, step-by-step.

main uncomfortable, and swelling may occur in the calf area after excessive walking. Our follow-up investigations indicate that these problems can generally be caused to disappear spontaneously over a period of two to three months by resolutely following a program of medical exercise. Massage therapy can also be applied where there is some recurrence of symptoms or residual symptoms after surgical treatment; in these cases it will tend to improve the symptoms or cause them to vanish altogether. During the application of massage therapy, special attention should be paid to those patients who have suffered from hypertension. When blood pressure is running abnormally high, massage treatment should be suspended.

Our use of massage therapy to treat this condition is constantly improving, as we feel our way ahead. When we began, the results were not out of the ordinary. Between February 1959 and January 1962, we treated 131 cases. Of these, 51 cases (38.9 percent) recovered completely; 28 cases (21.4 percent) showed obvious improvement; 45 cases (34.4 percent) were somewhat improved; 7 cases (5.3 percent) showed no effect.

Therapeutic effect was raised after clinical experimentation with nearly 1000 cases allowed us to improve our massage techniques. New methods were invented and the degree of force used in massage was increased. Between April 1967 and January 1969, we treated 344 cases. Of these, 267 (77.6 percent) recovered completely; 29 (8.4 percent) showed obvious improvement; 35 (10.2 percent) showed some improvement; 13 (3.8 percent) showed no effect.

Between April 1969 and March 1971 we offered medical and health services to farmers in rural villages. One medical team found that 49 of the 53 cases they treated recovered completely. Two cases showed obvious improvement, one showed some improvement, and on one patient the treatment had no effect.

The therapeutic effect of massage therapy in treating this condition is affected by the following circumstances:

a) *The stage at which treatment is begun:* In acute cases within a few days of onset, several treatments usually bring recovery, with no residual symptoms. Where the condition has existed for months or even years, it can still be cured, but the number of treatments is correspondingly greater. In this situation some residual symptoms may remain.

Case History No. 1

Wang ———, male, age 22, a medical student. Low back pain and radiating pain in his right leg occurred suddenly several hours before, while he was working. While he was carrying a heavy object during the course of his work,

---

Standards of therapeutic effect

Recovery: The patient's symptoms completely disappeared. His physical signs returned to normal or near-normal. The legs could be elevated to 80 degrees or more. The patient could resume his original work.

Obvious improvement: Here the patient's symptoms were obviously improved, and only some symptoms remained. Generally, the patient's daily activities were not affected. His physical signs were also clearly improved. The straight-leg elevation reached approximately 70 degrees. The patient still found it difficult to participate in heavy work, and needed an appropriately reduced level of work.

Improvement: Here the patient's symptoms grew better. There was either no effect on his daily activities, or only slight inconvenience. His physical signs were improved, and the straight-leg elevation reached less than 70 degrees. The patient could not take part in heavy manual labor.

No effect: No change in symptoms and physical signs.

---

his lumbar area turned to the left, and he felt pain in his lower back, radiating down to his right calf and lateral condyle of the ankle. He could not bend his back and when he coughed the pain was aggravated. He had low back pain but no radiating pain in his medical history. In examination a tender pressure point was discovered beside his fourth and fifth vertebrae. The lumbar muscles were tense. A straight-leg elevation test produced lumbar pain at 45° on the right side and 60° on the left side. There was a numb area in the posterolateral aspect of the right calf. The reflex of the right Achilles tendon was weakened. An x-ray of the lumbar vertebrae did not show any signs of abnormality.

A diagnosis was made of "slipped disk" between the fourth and fifth lumbar vertebrae. Consequently, the previously described massage therapy was performed. After the first massage session the low back pain was immediately lessened and the extent of the mobility of the lumbar area was increased. The right leg could be elevated to 60 degrees and the left leg to 70 degrees. After the third massage session the low back pain had completely disappeared.

After the eighth session, all the symptoms completely vanished. Both legs could be elevated to 90 degrees. After a period of three months a visit was made to the patient. He was found participating in his normal studies and labor, with no symptoms remaining.

Case History No. 2

Yu ———, female, age 23, worker. She twisted her back while lifting up a heavy object. This resulted in low back pain and pain radiating into her right leg which she suffered for a whole day. Coughing and walking both caused pain. In examination her lumbar area was found to be flat, with no lateral curvature of the spinal column. There was a pressure pain at the level of the fifth lumbar intervertebral space, to the right side of the paravertebral muscles. The left leg could be elevated 90 degrees; the right leg, 35 degrees. The test involving bending back the big toes proved the right side to be weakened. A diagnosis was made of "slipped" fifth lumbar intervertebral disk. After the two massage sessions the symptoms disappeared. The patient was advised to take two weeks' rest before resuming her work. On a follow-up visit to her, we found she had returned to work, and that no symptoms remained.

b) *The extent of pathological change:* We came to a point where the treatment of seven of our cases had been without effect. Surgery was then used in five of these cases. During surgery pathologic changes were discovered, all fairly obvious. In four of these cases, there were big protrusions, and fibrosis of the tissues of the protruded intervertebral disk was fairly great. In one case, fairly serious adhesions had resulted outside the spino-meningeal canal and beside the nerve root. In still another case, although the patient was improving, he was nevertheless operated upon because his daily life and work were still affected. During the operation, it was discovered that there was a bilateral protrusion, as well as that pathological changes had taken place involving the formation of an annular scar that restricted the outside of the spino-meningeal canal. From these examples, it can be seen that the degree of pathologic change will greatly influence the effectiveness of the therapy.

c) *The appropriateness of the massage techniques:* The same methods cannot be used in all cases. If they are, it will have a direct effect on the success of the treatment. Case Histories 3 and 4 provide illustrations:

Case History No. 3

Lü ———, male, age 27. A month before, after wrenching his back while carrying a heavy object, he suddenly felt pain in the lower back and radiating pain in his left leg. When he bent his back, or coughed, the pain was aggravated. He was hospitalized in May. Examination found pressure pain in the paravertebral muscles on the left side of the fourth and fifth lumbar vertebrae. The left leg could be raised 30 degrees, the right 60 degrees. The test involving bending back the big toes showed that the left side was weakened. In the hospital the usual massage techniques were applied. At times the symptoms were improved, at times they became worse. After about a month of treatment no satisfactory result had been achieved; no apparent increase in straight-leg elevation was observed. On 20 June of the same year, the cause for the ineffectiveness of the therapy was investigated. It was found that the patient's main difficulty was in bending forward. As a result the use of the lumbar stretch method was changed so that more backward extension was done, and the lower-limb stretch technique was added. The symptoms completely vanished after ten days of treatment. The straight-leg elevation of both legs returned to normal. Medical exercise was prescribed as well, in order to consolidate the treatment. After ten days of this, the patient had recovered and left the hospital.

Case History No. 4

Wang ———, male, age 29, rural cadre. Two weeks before hospitalization he was suddenly attacked by low back pain and radiating pain in the left lower leg. Because he had made a long journey on foot across mountains and rivers, he was exhausted, and suffered an attack of lumbar pain. Over the past three years he had a history of intermittent lumbar pain. This most recent occurrence was the most severe: the pain radiated down to the back of the knee of the left leg and there was a feeling of numbness on the outside of the calf. Walking less than 100 meters caused the pain in his lower back and leg to increase, and made him limp. In examination a pressure pain area was discovered in the paravertebrae on the left side of the fourth and fifth vertebrae. The left leg could be elevated to 30 degrees. The muscles of the left calf were rather loose and soft. An x-ray was consonant with the pathology of protrusion of an intervertebral disk. Protrusion of a lumbar intervertebral disk was diagnosed. After applying the aforementioned massages 3–4 times, lumbar pain disappeared and straight-leg elevation also approached normal. But a sore, swelling pain remained in the left ilium and buttocks. The lumbar stretch and lower-limb stretch methods were not continued. In addition to medical exercise, more rubbing and rolling of the lumbar, buttock, and iliac areas was applied. After 20 days the symptoms had completely disappeared, and he left the hospital.

d) *Other treatment:* There can be definite additional benefit in combining other treatment arrangements with massage, where conditions permit. And in acute cases, therapeutic results are better when complete bed rest is possible during the course of treatment. The most difficult cases to treat are those in which the fifth lumbar intervertebral disk is protruded. In such cases, care must be taken to select the appropriate methods of treatment.

Lastly, based on the understanding acquired in our clinical work, here are some preliminary ideas about the principles involved in massage treatment of this condition:

a) *The reducing action of massage techniques:* In massage treatment of this condition, passive manipulations such as the lumbar stretch method are used. This is because their kinetic action on the spinal column causes the tissues of the protruded intervertebral disk to return to their original position. This may be one of the most important principles in the massage treatment of slipped disk. The fact that the symptoms were largely alleviated after one treatment in the cases of acute injury described above helps to demonstrate this point. Another example is given below:

Case History No. 5

Shao ———, male, 25 years of age. Through examination and medical history the disease was definitely diagnosed as protrusion of a lumbar intervertebral disk. A laminotomy was performed, and the protrusion was removed. A round, elastic protruded nodule of 1×0.5 cm was observed in the lateral antero-superior part of the first sacral nerve, after the disk tissue between the dextral lumbar 5 and the sacral 1 vertebrae was exposed. The lumbar stretch method was then applied. When the hip was bent forward, the distance between the lumbar 5 and the sacral 1 spinous processes became larger; as the leg was extended backward, this gap reached and passed normal, finally becoming a narrow slit. After applying this massage method five times, the protruded nodule completely disappeared. Examination of the protruded area with a neuro-stripper showed that its elasticity had also returned to normal.

The above example shows that passive manipulation can reduce the intervertebral disk tissue to its original condition. However, in some already chronic cases a longer time is required before reduction is achieved.

Case History No. 6

Zhang ———, female, 19 years of age. Protrusion of the lumbar 5 sacral 1 intervertebral disk was diagnosed prior to surgery. The condition had already existed for six months. Massage therapy was tried six times in the outpatient department, without success. Then she was operated on. During the operation, in the middle of the nerve root, toward its medial side, a protruded object of rather high tension was found. The lumbar stretch method was applied eight times, but the protruded object did not shrink back. And examination with a neuro-stripper clearly showed that its tension had not lessened. The protruded object was then extracted. When the nucleus pulposus was scraped away the protruded object was found to have degenerated into a frozen mass without fluidity.

The foregoing example illustrates the fact that when the nucleus pulposus has already degenerated it is not likely to be possible to reduce a protruded disk with one application of massage. If the pathologic changes in the disk are even more severe, even a long course of massage will not return them to normal.

b) Loosening adhesions: It is generally conceded that massage has the effects of loosening local adhesions in the tissues near an injury, relieving inflammation of the nerves and freeing the nerve roots. But massage also has the effects of stopping pain, improving circulation, reducing swelling, and clearing away extravasated blood.

In our clinical observations we found that in almost all chronic cases the effect of massage was not manifested at an early stage in the treatment. However, where the massage was maintained over a fairly long period of time, its therapeutic effect gradually became heightened. With this in mind, we conclude that the lower-limb stretch method may have the effect of freeing the nerve roots from surrounding adhesions. We also observed that during intervertebral disk surgery, when the straight-leg elevation test was done, the nerve roots in the intervertebral space moved. Applications of the lower-limb stretch method, in cases where there was no pain, resulted in a gradual increase in the height of straight-leg elevation. This indicates the possibility that the lower-limb stretch gradually pulls apart adhesions of the nerve roots. In some cases symptoms remained after surgery, and these could often be treated by massage therapy. In a number of cases, the postoperative symptoms were probably caused by postoperative adhesions. Therefore, we see that massage can be used to treat postoperative symptoms. This helps to illustrate the use of massage in loosening adhesions.

Case History No. 7

Wu ———, male, age 34, rural cadre. For seven years he had complained of pain in the lumbar region and right leg, resulting from falling off a horse. As a result, he entered the hospital for medical examination. By x-ray studies of the nucleus pulposus, a prolapse between the 4th and 5th lumbar intervertebral disks were confirmed. His operation was on the 15th of April. Postoperative symptoms remained of radiating pain in the right leg, with a numb sensation on the outside of the calf. The right leg was elevated 35 degrees; the left leg 50 degrees. Twenty days after the operation the incision had healed well but the symptoms did not show any sign of improvement. Massage therapy was immediately begun. After the fourth massage session the pain he had complained of in his leg, and the numb sensation as well had both been mitigated. Straight-leg elevation of the right leg was increased to 60 degreees; of the left leg to 80 degrees. After the massage had been applied eleven times the pain and numbness in the leg had completely vanished. Straight-leg elevation on the right side was 80 degrees; on the left, 85 degrees. However, the strength of the back muscles was fairly poor. Massage was stopped and the patient was instructed in medical exercise. He was told to continue the exercises after he left the hospital.

c) *Other functions:* Local kneading and rolling can relieve pain, relax excess tension in the muscles and prevent muscle strain or atrophy. The lumbar rotation method has a positive effect on deformities of the lumbar vertebrae and helps improve the body's compensatory powers. The lower-limb stretch may also be conducive to eliminating the pathological lesion that gave rise to the pain in the affected leg.

2. Rheumatoid Spondylitis

Rheumatoid spondylitis is a particularly conspicuous type of pathologic change of the spinal column in rheumatoid arthritis. Pathologic changes attack all the tissues that constitute the joints, resulting finally in stiffness and deformation. The doctor of Chinese traditional medicine regards it as a type of paralysis and divides it into three different forms: walking paralysis, aching paralysis, and localized paralysis. Wind, cold, and moisture, the so-called three external evils, are thought to attack the body, giving rise to the disease. Walking paralysis is caused by wind, aching paralysis by cold, and localized paralysis by moisture.

Etiology

The actual cause of the disease is not yet completely known. We only know that some factors are definitely related to its occurrence. Some cases break out following symptoms such as those of the common cold, tonsillitis, or sinusitis. The bodies of some patients contain chronic infective foci such as tonsillitis or caries of the teeth. Some cases are considered to be connected with streptococcal infection, because the agglutinin titre of streptococcus haemolyticus in the patient's blood serum is high. Sometimes, trauma near a joint causes a drop in its resistance to infection, allowing rheumatoid arthritis to set in. People who are rather tense or who worry constantly are also susceptible to the disease. Living and working in a damp environment and being attacked by wind, cold, and moisture also have a definite relation with the disease.

Symptoms

In a minority of cases, the symptoms of rheumatoid spondylitis break out in an acute form following a cold. These symptoms include fever and aching soreness over the whole body. Most important is that all or part of the spinal column is very sore, there is difficulty in turning over, and the neck is sore and cannot be turned. In the majority of cases, however, development is slow and chronic. There is soreness in the vertebral region, either fixed in a certain location or wandering. When the weather is changeable, such as during generally cloudy, rainy weather, the pain increases. It comes and goes, but never entirely clears up. Gradually, hypoactivity of the vertebral column develops. The spine will not bend forward or backward and its sideways movement also becomes limited. Because of this, there is an obvious decline in the ability to put on clothes or shoes, to bend the lumbar region, to pick things up off the floor, etc. It finally develops into the deformities of lumbar curvature and hunch-back, and the patient cannot sit long, carry heavy loads, or lie flat. Normal daily actions become difficult and ability to work declines. At the same time, because the joints between the ribs and the vertebrae are attacked and their movement interfered with, the ability to breathe is affected. In its late stages the disease is accompanied by anemia, anorexia, dizziness, insomnia, and psychasthenia — manifestations of systemic weakness. Another feature is that the disease often occurs in manhood.

Diagnosis

Because it is difficult to diagnose the disease in its early stages, it is often missed. It is easier to diagnose in its later stages, on the basis of the symptoms outlined above. Enumeration and classification of the leucocytes and blood sedimentation will help to identify the developmental condition of the pathologic changes. For accurate diagnosis, X-ray photography is the best method. Exposures must be made of the front and side of the aching vertebral column. Sometimes it is necessary to include both sides of the sacroiliac and the hip joints. On the x-ray the special features of rheumatoid spondylitis can be seen. Generally, calcium deposits at the small joints of the spinal column are evident, as well as bony proliferation on the margins of the vertebral body. Hence the articular space may become hazy. In typical cases, the spinal column takes on the so-called "bamboo-section" or "waterfall" appearances.

Treatment

This is a kind of chronic disease. In the course of treatment tell the patient clearly about his condition and what result application of the proper massage therapy can achieve. Close cooperation between the doctor and the patient is an important factor in assuring that the treatment is effective. In fact, it is the severely ill patient who resolutely carries out his own therapy, by means of massage and directed medical exercise, who can take a turn for the better and regain his power of movement.

a) Massage: (i) Normally, the prone position is used, with the chest and abdomen cushioned by pillows of the proper height. If the pathologic changes are chiefly located on the upper part of the back, or if the patient's back is too stiff for him to lie prone, then a sitting position is used.

(ii) First apply the flat-thumb push method on either side of the spinal column, and then do a circular rubbing of the back with the thumbs, or apply the palm-rub method or the dig method on the same area. Go from top to bottom and bottom to top, back and forth for ten minutes or so.

(iii) Apply acupoint massage: If the pathologic changes are mainly located in the upper part of the back or in the neck area, then use the *fengchi, fengfu, jianjing,* and *dazhui* points. If the pathologic changes are chiefly located in the lumbar and the hip areas, then the *shenshu, mingmen,* eight *liao,* and *huantiao* massage points can be used. Apply the finger-dig, finger-vibrate and thumb-tip push methods on all the points mentioned.

The massage is applied chiefly to relax the muscles, increase circulation of the blood, and strengthen the body's resistance.

(iv) Based on the site of the pathologic degeneration, various types of rotation and stretching exercises are adopted. In the treatment of this disease, these are the key to restoring the ability to move. In performing such techniques, skillful use must be made of a number of different positions. For neck rotation or lumbar rotation, a sitting position is recommended; for steady pressing on the vertebral column, a prone position; for hip rotation and stretching the lower limbs, a supine position. In performing the various types of motion technique, the important thing is to gradually turn and pull out the ankylosed joints. In our practical experience, we have found that articular ankylosing is not something absolute, but resembles the situation when chains winding round the axle of a windlass become rusted to a state of immobility. If the proper amount of force is applied to the "rusted" joint, then the joint can gradually be loosened. However, the degree of loosening each time should not be too great. The use of force in therapeutic manipulation must be properly handled. Enough strength should be used each time to achieve a little loosening, as long as the patient can stand it. If too much force were used, not only would the patient not be able to stand the pain, but joint hemorrhage and swelling would occur, even to the point of evoking the reaction of high fever etc. Moreover, it would affect the progress of the treatment.

(v) Different conditions of the disease require different treatments. When pathologic degeneration is in an active stage, and the patient has severe pain, fever, and high hematic sedimentation, push and rub massage of the back and massage of the acupoints can be the basis of treatment, in order to strengthen the patient's constitution. When the pathologic degeneration mainly involves ankylosis, various kinds of passive manipulation are applied, to free the ankylosed joints. A patient's condition is usually compound, however, so various techniques must be skillfully combined. Some ankylosed cases are in a very critical condition, close to paralysis. In these cases, a step-by-step plan must be devised to solve the problems one at a time. In cases where most of the joints in the body are ankylosed, the most important problem must be solved first. Usually, the coxal joint is freed first, restoring the patient's ability to walk. Then the problem of restoring movement to the joints in the vertebral spines is addressed.

b) Other treatment: Some hormones such as prednisone tablets etc., taken orally, can be used in treatment of the active-phase patient. But at the chronic stage, physical therapies such as electro-therapy and hydrotherapy can be combined with the massage or the proper Chinese herbal medicine can be used. If the disease becomes more severe during the winter, and the patient shows a tendency to feel the cold, the following herbs can be used:

Shudi	3 liang	Rehmannia glutinosa (steamed root)
Shouwu	3 liang	Polygonum multiflorum Thunb. (root)
Congrong	3 liang	Cistanche deserticola
Fuzi	1 liang	Aconitum carmichaeli Debx. (root)
Xiangfu	3 liang	Cyperus rotundus L. (rhizome)
Yanhusuo	3 liang	Corydalis yanhusuo (rhizome)
Qinjiao	3 liang	Gentiana macrophylla (root)
Mugua	3 liang	Chaenomeles lagenaria Koidz. (fruit)
Danggui	3 liang	Angelica sinensis (root)
Chenpi	2 liang	Orange or tangerine peel

The herbs are ground into powder and rolled together into sugar-coated pellets. Dosage is 3 *qian*, twice a day.

In order to consolidate the effectiveness of the massage and to promote restoration of articular function, medical exercises must be started early in the course of treatment.

Therapeutic effect

Massage has been found satisfactory in treating this disease. The aching becomes somewhat worse during the first few days of treatment, then gradually improves. Step by step, articular and respiratory function can be improved or restored. Pain is mitigated to the same degree that articular movement is restored. Muscular atrophy and muscular strength can both gradually be improved. Appetite and general condition also improve by degrees. Treatment of this disease by massage therapy does take a comparatively long time, about three to six months. But as long as medical exercise is maintained over a long period, not only can the therapeutic effect be solidified, but function can continue to improve.

Case History No. 1

Zhou ———, male, age 33, cadre in an organization. Came to the hospital for treatment in February. For eight or nine years he had experienced pains in the hip and knee, and the spinal column. The pain came and went with rainy weather and was most likely to appear in spring and autumn. He had been through various treatments, but all were in vain. Lately the pains had been occurring frequently. Movement of the vertebral column was obviously obstructed and when walking he showed lumbar curvature and hunch-back. In examination, with his spinal column bent forward, the tips of his fingers only reached his knees and he could not bend low enough to put his shoes on. The vital capacity of his lungs was only 2450 ml. X-rays showed the specific features of rheumatoid spondylitis: the thoracic-lumbar section of the spinal column already displayed "bamboo-section" and "waterfall" degeneration. There were aching and swelling reactions after the first two massage therapy sessions, but from then on his condition gradually improved. After half a month he felt better, the pain was reduced and spinal movement was freer. After three months of massage therapy the pains had completely disappeared. Only on dark, rainy days did slight pain occasionally set in. The mobility of

Medical Exercise

(i) *Chest lift:* As in the treatment of prolapsed lumbar intervertebral disk (see Diagram 64, p. 95).

(ii) *Backward leg extension:* From a prone position, extend the left leg backward and upward, the higher the better, straightening the knee (see Diagram 68). Lower the legs after maintaining the highest position for a half a minute. Alternate left and right legs, doing each one 20–40 times.

DIAGRAM 68

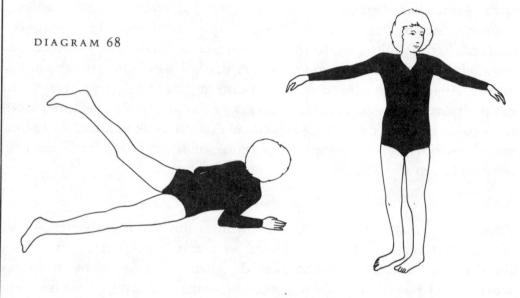

DIAGRAM 69

(iii) *Lumbar turn:* Stand with the feet set shoulder-width apart and the arms held up evenly to each side. Turn the neck and the waist as far to one side as possible. The motion should not be fast, but a full effort must be made to turn as far as possible (see Diagram 69). First turn left, then right. Repeat the process 20–50 times.

the vertebral column was greatly enlarged. When he bent forward, the tips of his fingers reached 15 cm below the knees. He could bend his lumbar vertebrae to pick up things from the ground, and to put on his shoes. The vital capacity of his lungs reached 2900 ml. New x-rays showed no further degeneration. After six months of treatment, the aching had altogether vanish-

(iv) *Lumbar bend:* Stand with feet set shoulder-width apart. Keeping the legs straight, bend forward at the waist, bouncing gradually forward until the hands touch the ground (see Diagram 66, p. 95). Then do the backward lumbar extension (see Diagram 67, p. 95). Then do lateral lumbar bends to the left and right (see Diagram 70). Require the patient to gradually bend his waist further and further. Bend 20–30 times in each direction.

(v) *Sand-bag exercise:* Suitable for the patient with no strength in the muscles of the lower limbs. The patient lies supine. Make a linen bag to contain about 20 catties[1] of sand. Start with 7–8 catties. Attach the bag to the patient's ankle, having him straighten out his leg and lift the sand-bag (see Diagram 71). The lifting should be repeated 10 times. If the patient can raise his leg more than 16 times, then the weight is not heavy enough and more sand should be added. If he can raise it fewer than 6 times, the weight is too heavy and the amount of sand should be reduced. Alternate legs and do each leg about 60 times. As function improves, gradually increase the weight of the bag.

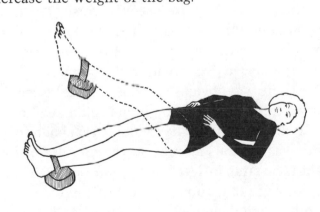

DIAGRAM 70   DIAGRAM 71

ed and the vertebral column moved even more freely. Therefore, the therapy was stopped. Inquiry two years later showed that his condition had remained the same, with no further outbreaks of the disease.

---

1. 1 catty = 10 *Liang* = 17.6 ounces (1.1 lbs) = 500 g.

Case History No. 2

Wang ———, male, age 51, cadre of an organization. He had had an aching in the neck area for seven or eight years. Overwork and cloudy, humid weather caused his neck-pains to suddenly become excruciating. His neck became stiff; he could not move his head and when he did, the pain became worse. The pain was so intense that it affected his sleep. Examination: Body temperature was normal; the neck muscles were tense and sore to the touch; the head could only turn about 15 degrees. X-rays showed that it was rheumatoid spondylitis: pathologic degeneration was evident in the fourth, fifth, and sixth cervical vertebrae. After the first massage therapy session, he suddenly felt warm and comfortable, the pain was greatly allayed, and he could turn his head from side to side. After ten sessions the aching had completely disappeared and the mobility of the neck had returned to normal. An inquiry three months later showed no recurrence of the symptoms.

Case History No. 3

Xu ———, male, age 40, cadre. Came for treatment in October. Pains in the lower back, shoulders, and back had been present for about 10 years. Over the past three years they had become worse. The lumbar spines and hips gradually became ankylotic. Gradually, he lost the ability to walk and had to support himself with two canes. Movement was extremely difficult; he was almost paralyzed. Examination: It was found that his general health was still good. There was obvious ankylosis in the vertebrae of the lumbar area and in the two hip joints. The hip joints could bend to about 90 degrees but could not extend backward. They adducted at about 5 degrees and could not abduct. There was obvious atrophy in the muscles of the lower limbs. Supine, he could raise straight legs a little, but not against resistance. (X-rays showed obvious signs of rheumatoid anthritis in the low-back vertebral column, the sacroiliac, and the hip joints. Through the first few massage therapy sessions, the pain increased, but after about half a month, it began to get better. The intensity of the passive manipulation was gradually increased, so that the articular ankylosis was gradually freed. Although there was some painful reaction to each treatment, the patient stubbornly maintained his program of medical exercise, actively participating in the treatment. After about seven or eight months, the pain and the ankylosis were both gone and he could walk easily. Finally, he returned to work.

3. Lumbar Strain

Lumbar strain is a chronic type of condition frequently seen among working people, especially thsoe engaged in heavy labor requiring bending of the lumbar area or carrying heavy loads. For example many foundry-workers suffer from this problem.

Etiology

The ligaments and muscles around the lumbar vertebrae have not healed completely, or are continually being injured; there is no history of acute injurics, but the general constitution is comparatively weak. There are also those individuals engaged in heavy physical labour who cannot compensate for abnormalities originally existing in the spinal column. All these conditions can result in this condition.

However, there are some patients with good constitutions and no acute traumatic history in whom this condition sets in gradually due to long-term over-bending of the lower back, or the carrying of heavy loads on the back. This is also known as "occupational strain."

Symptoms

Pain in the lower back is the essential symptom of this disease. It mostly happens in the middle of the lower lumbar spinal column. It can also often produce aching on either side of the spinal column and on the iliac crest. Sometimes the pain is intense, at other times it is light. Generally, the pain is light in the morning and heavy in the evening. It is aggravated by long sitting, by overtiredness, or by damp weather. When the symptoms are severe, the patient has difficulty doing any labour, and even sitting up or turning over in bed may be difficult. Sleep and appetite are also affected.

Diagnosis

A preliminary diagnosis may be made based on etiology and symptoms. A careful local palpation should be done to detect whether there is a hard mass in the muscle, to test the extent of muscular tension, and to find out whether there is any definite point of pressure pain and to define the extent of such pain. At the same time, care must be taken to distinguish lumbar pain due to other causes. If the pain is caused by chronic inflammation of the pelvic cavity, the application of massage therapy will have little effect. Massage is contraindicated where the pain is due to inflammatory degeneration, such as in vertebral tuberculosis, etc. Where necessary, an x-ray should be taken to help eliminate other pathological changes as the cause of the pain and to make a definite diagnosis.

Treatment

a) Massage: Normal methods and sequence—

(i) The patient lies prone; his hands are placed on either side of his body. One or more pillows are placed under his abdomen, and all muscles are allowed to relax. First, the palm rub method is applied, starting from the pain-free part of the back and gradually progressing to the painful area. The manipulations should be applied lightly, so as not to cause pain, but to make the massaged area comfortable.

(ii) Next, the palm-heel kneading method or the roll method is employed, with a gradual increase of intensity, on either side of the spinal column, going up or down several times.

(iii) Third, with the thumb, deep kneading is applied to the main site of pain. It can simultaneously be combined with other methods such as the finger dig, the finger vibrate and the thumb kneading methods. Using all these methods, massage can be applied to such acupoints as *shenshu, mingmen* and the eight *liao (shangliao, zhongliao,* etc.). The thumb-tip push method is also used. Also, acupoint massage can be applied to the principal pressure pain sites.

(iv) Finally, at the conclusion of the massage, the kneading and the roll methods are again applied. At the same time the rotation and bend methods for the lower limbs can be performed lightly.

Methods for specific applications: (i) When the disease is caused by a chronic lesion of the interspinous ligaments, the pain is often confined to a certain spinous process or inter-vertebral space right in the middle of the spine. The pain occurs with the forward-bending, or backward-extending of the spine and there is a fixed local tender point. Stress should be placed on the thumb kneading and thumb-tip push methods, which are applied to the immediate painful area. The force of the thumb should gradually penetrate deeply into the painful area and from there one should push outward into the surrounding area.

(ii) If the condition is the result of a chronic lesion of the lumbar muscles, most of the pain will be in the lower part of the muscles at the sacral vertebrae or in the upper attachments of the lumbar muscles. Muscle-tension on one or both sides is often hyperactively great. There is pain when the spine is bent forward and the sides of the body are moved. A swollen mass or hard lump can sometimes be found in the soft tissues. When massaging the muscles, the kneading and roll methods should be used most. The thumb kneading method is employed on the site of the pain or the swollen mass. At a later stage, the energy-system pluck method can also be used. The kneading and rolling should be combined with rotation and stretching of the lower limbs.

(iii) If there is no history of external injury, and the strain of the lumbar muscles is due only to spinal deformity or over-tiredness in the lumbar region, and if the patient's lumbar muscles show the pathological changes associated with fasciitis, there will usually be obvious soreness in the lumbar area, as well as high muscle-tension and pressure-pain over a comparatively large area. Massage should be light. In the local area, the rub, kneadng, and roll methods are used. Acupoint massage is also important. Besides the *jianyu*, *mingmen*, and eight *liao* acupoints, distant acupoints on the lower limbs, such as *chengfu*, *weizhong*, *chengshan* and *taixi* can be used.

b) *Other Treatment:* In addition to massage, physical therapy, acupuncture, and herbal fomentations can also be used. If the condition is due to spinal deformity or weakness of the lumbar muscles, medical exercise should be used as well. Programs of exercise may be used that either correct the deformity or strengthen the lumbar muscles. Both of these will help to heighten and consolidate therapeutic effect.

Therapeutic effect

The therapeutic effect of massage therapy on lumbar strain will be greatly affected by the pathological process by which the strain was formed, and the duration of the condition. Generally speaking, massage therapy is effective in treating this condition. (For treatment by massage therapy of lumbar strains ensuing from bone injuries or spinal deformity, see the section on Other Chronic Lumbar Pain following.) Some patients may suffer recurrences which must be guarded against. This is especially so in the case of occupational lumbar strain. Preventive measures are discussed below.

Case History

Fang ——————, male, age 37, cadre. The patient had suffered lumbar pain for two or three years. There was no history of trauma and the pain appeared

---

Medical Exercise for Prevention of Lumbar Strain

(i) *Chafing the lumbus:* Done standing or in the normal working position. With the radial sides of both fists (the "eyes" of the fists) chafe upwards with force along both sides of the lumbar spine. Do 50–200 strokes each time, chafing until the lumbar region feels warm. When using the normal working position, one can slowly straighten up into a standing position at the same time. Once standing straight, continue until the required warmth and number of strokes are reached.

(ii) *Extending the lumbus:* Similar to the movements involved in extending a "tired waist." Stand with feet shoulder-width apart. Raise both hands, at the same time breathing in, distending the abdomen, extending the waist backwards as far as possible and tensing all the muscles of the body. Then lower the hands to their original position, breathe out, and relax. Repeat several times.

(iii) *Bending at the waist:* Described in the medical exercises for protrusion of a lumbar intervertebral disk. See Diagram 66.

(iv) *Straightening the waist:* Take the archer's position, with the right leg a stride forward, the right hand pressing down on the right thigh, and the left hand supporting the left side of the lumbar area. Lower the body's centre of gravity, pushing on the lumbar area with the left hand and pressing down on the knee cap with the right hand. Lean backward from the waist, facing upwards, and push backward elastically several times, gradually increasing the range of movement. Switch right and left legs and hands and repeat. Alternate, doing it each way 4–8 times. Lower the body's centre of gravity, press on the lumbar area with the left hand, press down on the knee with the right hand, and bend the upper body, backward. Repeat several times in a loose, rhythmic manner, gradually increasing the amount that the lumbar region bends. Then perform the same motions with the left leg forward and the right hand pushing on the lumbar region. Do it each way 4–8 times.

---

when he was fatigued. For the previous two months, the outbreaks had been more severe. The pain was aggravated by long sitting or standing and it affected sleep. Oral medication was ineffective. On examination there was a hard lump the size of a walnut and sore to the touch in the muscles on the left side of the lumbar area. An x-ray of the lumbar region showed no pathological changes in the bone. A diagnosis of lumbar strain was made.

After four sessions of the massage therapy described above, the patient felt that his pain was improving. After two weeks of treatment, the pain was reduced to the point that sleep was no longer affected. After 40 massage sessions, the pain was basically gone and the hard lump was clearly softened. The symptoms did not recur.

4. Other Chronic Lumbar Pain

Lumbar pain is an extremely common symptom. It can be symptomatic of a wide variety of conditions. In addition to protrusion of a lumbar intervertebral disk, lumbar strain and rheumatoid spondylitis, mentioned above, there are other causes of chronic lumbar pain such as obsolete and compressive fracture, and lumbo-sacralized or sacro-lumbarized megalo-spondylitis. Massage therapy has definite therapeutic effects in all of these. Because the massage therapy methods indicated are for the most part similar, these diseases are all described together below.

Etiology

In compressive fracture of the spine, there is generally a history of acute lesion. In the other diseases there is usually no obvious traumatic history, but just a slow development of the disease. The diseases are chiefly due to changes in the vertebral power line that cause retrogressive changes of a differing degree in the vertebral column. These affect normal physiological function, giving rise to lumbar pain.

Symptoms

The symptom common to these various conditions is chronic lumbar pain. It is often a persistent aching pain that occasionally becomes excruciating. Generally, the pain becomes more severe because of over-work or on gloomy, rainy days. It is usually located in the lumbar region, but some pains are referred to the back and some even appear in one or both of the sciatic nerves, leading to weakness in the lower limbs and numbness in the calf, etc. A protracted illness can affect systemic function as well as the ability to work.

Diagnosis

A preliminary diagnosis is made on the basis of the patient's history and symptoms. During examination, external anomalies of the lumbar region can often be discovered. The manifestations of this are that the lumbar section of the vertebral column is flat and even, and that the normal anteriorly convexed physiological arch becomes weakened or disappears. Some patients may have lateral spinal curvature. A definitive diagnosis may be made and the site and degree of the pathologic changes understood by means of x-rays.

Treatment

a) *Massage:* (i) The patient is in a prone position. The chest and abdominal areas are padded with pillows. Apply the rub, kneading, and roll methods to relax the paravertebral muscles.

(ii) The thumb-push and roll methods are used in deep massage, concentrating on the aching areas. The thumb-push, finger-dig, and finger-vibrate methods are applied to the acupoints that correspond to the aching areas and at the site of the pain.

(iii) Passive movement of the lumbar area: As a rule, a forceful backward-extension is used (see Diagram 46, p. 47). No great force is needed, but the extension should be repeated about 10 to 20 times. If there are symptoms of sciatica, then the slanting backward-extension method may be added. This procedure is repeated 5 or 6 times, using somewhat greater force for the last extension.

b) *Other treatment:* Other physical therapies may be used in conjunction with the massage therapy. The number of massage therapy sessions need not be too great — about 10 or 15. When the pain has lessened or disappeared, encourage the patient to undertake a long-term program of medical exercise lasting at least 3 to 6 months, to correct the shape of the spine and strengthen the paravertebral muscles.

Medical Exercise

(i) *Chest lift:* See medical exercises for protrusion of lumbar intervertebral disk, p. 94 and Diagram 64, p. 95.

(ii) *Backward extension of both legs:* The patient is in a prone position. The legs are drawn tightly together and extended straight. Try to keep the knees as straight as possible. Slowly lift both legs, the higher the better, and maintain them at their highest point for thirty seconds to a minute. The lumbar muscle will feel very tense and full of force. When this position can no longer be sustained, slowly lower the legs and rest for a while. Repeat a total of 5 to 10 times. (See Diagram 72).

(iii) *Jumping like a fish:* See medical gymnastics for protrusion of a lumbar intervertebral disk, p. 94 and Diagram 65, p. 95.

(iv) *Lumbar stretch:* The patient is in a standing position, with legs set shoulder-width apart and both hands supporting the lumbar area. With a gentle bouncing motion extend the waist forward and flatten the abdomen, repeating 30 to 60 times and gradually increasing the amount of extension.

(v) *Lumbar suspension:* With both hands, grasp a horizontal bar, such as the top of a door-frame, set just high enough that the toes can still touch the ground (see Diagram 73). Hanging half-suspended, swing the lower back loosely and naturally forward and backward, and from side to side. The breadth of the swing can gradually be increased to a point where the lumbar spines can rotate. Persist until the arms can no longer hang on, rest for a while and then repeat several times.

DIAGRAM 72   DIAGRAM 73

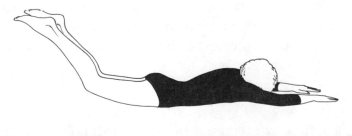

Therapeutic Effect

At the beginning of the therapy and medical gymnastics there may be severe lumbar pain. That this is normal should be explained to the patient before treatment. Explain clearly the importance of long-term medical exercise to consolidate and heighten the therapeutic effect, and encourage the patient to make a firm decision to stubbornly combat the condition.

Case History

Gao ———, male, age 42, cadre. Suffered from low back pain five to six years. Though no history of trauma, symptoms were gradually getting more severe. Over the past two years, they had given rise to bilateral sciatica. The right side was more serious. The right lower limb was numb, painful, and weak. Examination showed that the lumbar spine was flat and even, the lumbar muscles obviously atrophied. There were pressure pains on both sides of the paravertebral spinous muscles, especially in the lower lumbar area. A straight leg raise with his right leg, brought referred pain as he reached 50°. Reflexes of the right knee and right heel were all weaker than those on the left side. Lumbo-sacralization was seen on the x-rays and a false articulation had already formed on the right side. For the past two years, many treatments were tried to no avail. He wore a leather girdle around his waist and used a cane. After walking 300 yards (250 m) his legs became numb and painful and he could go no further. He had been unable to work for almost two years. After four treatments, he felt the numbness in his legs begin to fade. After eight treatments, the pains in the lumbar and leg areas were clearly improved, so that he could walk without a cane. Then he began a program of medical exercise, and was encouraged to take off his leather girdle. After 30 treatments all symptoms were completely eliminated. The lumbar muscles were remarkably strengthened and there was no reaction to walking a distance. After another 15 treatments, he recovered and left the hospital. He was encouraged to maintain his program of medical exercise in order to consolidate the therapeutic effect of the treatment.

5. Sprains

Massage therapy has a beneficial effect on soft tissue and this is especially apparent with sprains. There is a wide variety of sprains, including all acute disorders that result from a sudden wrenching or twisting. A description follows of the sprains in the sites with soft tissues, particularly involving a sudden overstretching of the ligament, or injury due to wrenching. The most commonly seen locations of sprain are described below.

SPRAIN OF THE ANKLE JOINT

The sprain of the ankle joint is seen frequently. Usually when referring to an ankle sprain the true meaning is an injury to the lateral malleolar ligament. It seldom occurs in the medial malleolar joint. The injury occurs because of an overstretching of the ankle joint that suddenly bends outward or inward beyond the physiological scope of the articular movement, thereby causing injury to the lateral malleolar ligament. The injuries associated with differing degrees of sprain can be divided into the over-tension of the ligament, its partial, and complete tearing away.

Etiology

This kind of injury most often occurs while walking on uneven ground, or jumping down from a height. Injury results from the foot suddenly bending outward or inward.

Symptoms

(i) Aching pains: When an injury occurs pain suddenly appears in the lateral (or medial) part of the ankle, becoming more severe while moving about, or carrying a heavy load.

(ii) Swelling: Because of localized hemorrhage and the effusion of tissue fluid, the injury at once results in swelling. Swelling is mostly partially confined to the antero-inferior part of the ankle.

(iii) Hematomatic area under the skin (bruising): This is caused by the localized rupture of a small blood vessel with the blood collecting under the skin. In more serious cases of sprain the hematomatic spot and the blueish-purple discoloration of the skin, are usually present in the antero-inferior part of the ankle.

(iv) Crippling: Generally a crippling reaction appears right after the injury.

Diagnosis

Diagnosis is easier where there is a history of trauma together with localized symptoms. The tender point should be checked in order to identify the main site of an injury and to arrive at a correct diagnosis. If necessary, an x-ray examination should be performed in order to exclude fracture and dislocation.

Treatment

In accordance with the principle of accelerating the removal of the hematoma, generating new blood, and facilitating the flow of vital energy and blood, massage therapy is best applied at the acute stage of sprain.

(a) Massage: (i) Apply a light push or a light rub massage around the sprained area.

(ii) Apply a heavy stimulating manipulation like the finger-dig method, or the finger-vibrate method, on the *juegu* acupoint (the space between the tibia and fibula) of the affected limb, and continue manipulating this area for one minute. This is called the pain-removing method.

(iii) The push, rub, and kneading methods are applied around the sprained area along the direction of the vein and lymphatic returns.

(iv) Adopt the light to gradually heavier push and rub massage techniques, moving gradually from the circumference to the center of the injured area. If swelling and circumscribed bruising are present, use the thumb to apply, alternately, the finger-cut and push methods lightly and smoothly and with a dense pattern of strokes to the swollen area where blood has accumulated (the bruised area). Push upward from the lower part of the ankle to the cruciate ligament, continuing until the swelling disappears.

(v) Immediately thereafter apply the finger-dig and finger-vibrate methods to massage points in the area of the injury, such as *juegu, chengshan, kuenlun, taixi, jiexi, pushen* (below the lateral malleoleus, about 2 *cun* directly beneath the *kunlun* cavity, the depression beside the calcaneus bone) and *rangu* (in the depression in front of the medial malleoleus and below the sphenoid bone). N.B. When the finger dig method is applied, go from shallow to deep until a reaction is produced, then add the vibrate method and go from deep to shallow.

Massage once a day for 10 to 15 minutes until all the symptoms are gone.

b) Other treatment: At the acute stage of sprain it is necessary to combine massage with external application of a Chinese herbal preparation for improving circulation of vital energy and blood.

The following 18 different herbs should be totally pulverized into fine powder. Mix a proper amount with warm water to make a paste; put on a piece of gauze, spread the gauze over the affected area and hold it evenly in place with a bandage. Cover from the instep to the upper part of the ankle. After massage use the same prescription in a plaster applied to the affected area.

Chuanwu	6 *qian*	Aconitum carmichaeli Debx. (root)
Caowu	6 *qian*	Aconitum chinense Pext. (root)
Baizhi	1 *liang*	Angelica anomala (root)
Xiaohuixiang	2 *liang*	Foeniculum vulgare Mil. (fennel; fruit)
Rougui	2 *liang*	Cinnamomum cassia Blume (bark)
Ruxiang	3 *liang*	Boswellia glabra (frankincense)
Moyao	3 *liang*	Commiphora myrrha Engler (myrrh)
Xuejie	3 *liang*	Daemonorops draco Blume (dragon's blood)
Qianghuo	3 *liang*	Notopterygium incisum Ting. (root)
Duhuo	3 *liang*	Angelica pubescens Maxim. (root)
Xiangfu	3 *liang*	Cyperus rotundus L. (rhizome)
Niuxi	3 *liang*	Achyranthes bidentata Bl. (root)
Xuduan	3 *liang*	Dipsacus japonicus Mig. (root)
Chuanxiong	3 *liang*	Ligusticum wallichii Franch (rhizome)
Chishao	3 *liang*	Paeonia lactiflora Pall.(red peony root)
Zirantong	3 *liang*	Native copper
Danggui	5 *liang*	Angelica sinensis (root)
Zijingpi	5 *liang*	Cercis chinensis Bge. (bark)

Case History

Wang ———, male, age 17, student. Landed carelessly during a jumping exercise, turning his right foot inward and spraining it. Swelling immediately occurred in the right ankle joint area. When he walked around the pain was aggravated. Simultaneously, a swollen numb sensation developed. The following day he came to the hospital for treatment. Examination showed that the circumference of the right ankle joint was obviously swollen, and the swelling had spread to the instep of the foot. A hematomatic spot was found on the medial malleolus. A tender point on the front part of the lateral malleolus, or at the attachment of the anterior talofibular ligament was clearly noticeable. He walked with a limp. Massage with an anti-swelling and pain-killing medicinal powder was given. After the first massage the swelling had distinctly subsided and the pain was alleviated. After three massages, and three administrations of Chinese herbal medicine, the swelling pain and the hematomatic spot had entirely disappeared. While walking he still experienced a slight, sore, swollen pain. After three further massages all symptoms completely disappeared. On a visit to him, no after-symptoms were found.

LUMBAR SPRAIN

Sprain in the lumbar region is seen frequently. It can be caused by several different types of injuries:

a) When the waist bends forward to the lumbar point at which the lumbar spine is completely bent, the muscle-contraction that protects the ligament is no longer possible. So when the upper body bears a weight, the ligament to the lumbar region is susceptible to injury.

b) When the lower limbs are in the extended position, i.e. when the pelvis is fixed, and an excessive tractive force is suddenly applied to the lumbar region, injury to the ligament results.

c) A blow to the lumbar region and a sudden twisting when lifting a heavy object are factors that can produce lumbar sprain directly. In addition to injury of the ligament, injury of the lumbar muscles is also likely to occur.

Etiology

Lumbar sprain can be brought on by working with a bent back, by falling while doing heavy physical labour, and especially by a sudden twist while lifting a heavy object up off the floor.

Symptoms

There is pain on one or both sides of the lumbar region, which can neither bend forward or backward nor turn left or right. In serious cases, the patient needs someone to support him while he walks, and the pain becomes worse when he takes a deep breath or coughs. The swelling is often not manifest. During examination let the patient lie prone with several pillows under his abdomen. Then, with light and careful finger-pressure, a local pressure point can be discovered on lumbar spine 4 or 5, or in the space between lumbar spine 5 and sacrum 1. Sometimes, when the tender area is extensive, simultaneous injury to the muscle should be considered.

Diagnosis

Diagnosis is not difficult when there is a traumatic history of bending the lumbar spine and carrying a heavy load in combination with the symptoms and physical signs mentioned above. However, protrusion of the lumbar intervertebral disk etc. must first be excluded.

Treatment

a) *Massage:* (i) The affected person is in a prone position. The light rub method or the thumb-push method is first applied to the lumbar region so as to relax the lumbar muscles and reduce the pain.

(ii) Apply the roll method to both sides of the lumbar area. The massage should be light. Then the thumb, or the palm and outside edge of the hand are employed to knead around the circumference of the injury, after a while working gradually in toward the middle. Slowly move from light kneading to deep kneading, in order to relax the muscles and enliven the blood, clearing away the accumulated blood and producing new blood. This procedure is repeated several times.

(iii) Acupoint massage. Use the kneading and dig techniques on sites in the lumbar region, and the *shenshu, mingmen, shangliao, ciliao, huantiao, chengfu,* and *weizhong* acupoints.

(iv) Press on the lumbar spine and shift the pelvis. With his right hand, the therapist lightly presses on the lumbar region and with his left hand he moves the right side of the pelvis upward. Go from top to bottom, co-ordinating each pressure on the lumbus with a shift of the pelvis.

(v) Strike the lumbar region with the palm. With a concave palm, slap the lumbar region ten times, or more.

(vi) With the patient on his feet, apply the kneading and lumbar stretch methods to the lumbar region. For more detailed information on the lumbar stretch method, see page 45. Massage once daily for 20–25 minutes until all the symptoms disappear.

b) *Other treatment:* Apply a fomentation of Chinese medicinal herbs to the affected area for 10 to 20 minutes after each massage. Other physical therapies can also be employed. The brick-swat method from Chinese folk-medicine is also effective in the treatment of this disease (see instructions below).

Case History

Yang ———, female, age 19, teacher. Two weeks previously when taking part in manual labour, she lifted a heavy object and suddenly twisted her lumbar spine. She felt immediate pain in the lumbar region and could neither bend forward nor straighten up. After a period of rest the mobility of the lumbar spine was slightly improved, but pain persisted on both sides of the lumbar region, so she came to the hospital for treatment. After the above massage was applied once, the pain was suddenly reduced and lumbar mobility improved considerably. After the four massage sessions, the symptoms completely disappeared and she recovered. A follow-up visit to her showed no residual symptoms.

The Chinese Folk Brick-Swat Method

The patient lies prone and extends the two lower limbs out straight, holding the muscles extremely tense. The feet extend beyond the end of the bed and a soft pillow is placed as padding between the instep and the edge of the bed. The doctor, standing on the patient's left side, uses his left hand to hold down the lower parts of the patient's calves and keep the patient's heels close together. With his right hand the doctor takes a brick, squarely knocking the bottoms of the patient's heels with it 3 to 5 times with some force. Be careful to use the flat of the brick and to strike the heels squarely. Make sure that the patient's knees are straight, allowing the impact to carry up to the lumbar region.

SPRAIN OF THE ACCESSORY LIGAMENTS OF THE KNEE

The knee joint is the big joint that gives the human body its ability to bear heavy loads. Its structure is rather complicated. The stability of the joint relies entirely upon support from the surrounding muscles and the accessory ligaments on both sides of it, as well as from the cruciform ligaments of the interior of the knee joint. Sprain of the medial ligament of the knee joint is most common. Because of the comparative strength of the lateral accessory ligament and the toughness of the iliotibial band that protects it, the lateral accessory ligament is not easily injured. Injury generally occurs when the calf suddenly shifts or rotates outward, or when the calf stays where it is and the thigh suddenly moves and rotates inward. These produce injury to the medial accessory ligament. Sudden inward motion of the calf may produce injury to the lateral accessory ligament.

Etiology

During a fall, the calf abducts or rotates outward to touch the ground. One falls with the calf in a mudhole. A blow is struck on the side of the knee. All these can bring about an injury to the medial ligament. This injury can happen easily during sporting activities, for example when an athlete lands badly after kicking a football or jumping over a box-horse.

Symptoms

There is often a sudden severe pain on the affected side of the wounded knee, and when the lateral accessory ligament is injured, a protective muscle spasm often appears, causing the knee joint to remain bent. During examination, an obvious pressure pain is present in the ligament area, leading to localized pain on the wounded side. The same kind of pain can also develop when a heavy load is imposed upon the knee.

Diagnosis

If there is no abnormal movement in the knee joint, the injury is a simple incomplete laceration of the medial or lateral accessory ligament. If there is abnormal movement, then the ligament is completely torn or severed. When the injury is severe, injury to the medial or lateral accessory ligament is often combined with injuries to the articular capsule, the meniscus and the cruciform ligament. These must all be carefully distinguished.

Treatment

Good results are obtained from early massage treatment of incomplete laceration of the medial or lateral accessory ligament. If it is completely avulsed or severed, then good results are not obtained with massage therapy. Severe cases need immobilization or surgery.

a) Massage: (i) The patient lies on his back. A pillow is placed under the knee of the wounded limb. First remove the pain by applying the dig technique on the *xuehai* massage point.

(ii) On the upper part of the swollen area, apply the thumb-push method followed immediately by the kneading method, going from the distal point to the proximal point.

(iii) apply the finger-cut method to the swollen and sensitive area going from the distal point to the proximal point until the swelling subsides. Then the palm kneading method is applied to the affected site.

(iv) The kneading and dig methods are applied to the *xiyan, yinlingquan, yanglingquan, weizhong* and *heding* acupoints.

(v) Apply passive manipulation, bending and extending the genual articulation in a gentle, deft manner. Do not use excessive force.

(vi) Finally, the knead and pinch method are applied to the muscles around the knee.

Massage once daily, about 15 minutes or so each time, until all the symptoms disappear.

b) Other treatment: Immediately after massage, firmly wrap the affected area with a poultice of Chinese herbs (see p. 121). Generally the Chinese herbal medicine only need to be applied three times. If necessary, the physical therapy can be added.

Case History

Zhang ———, female, aged 59, housewife. She complained that the previous day, while carrying her baby, she turned to the right, carelessly spraining her left knee. This resulted in local swelling, pain and difficulty in walking. Rest did not alleviate the symptoms, so she came to the hospital for treatment. On examination, the whole left knee was swollen, especially on the outside, which was painful to the touch as well. Walking and carrying a heavy load increased the pain. The methods of massage outlined above were immediately employed, with external application of a poultice of Chinese herbs affixed to the affected area. After two massage treatments she recovered. A follow-up visit to her found her ability to work completely restored.

Therapeutic effect in sprain

In the treatment of sprain, massage has good therapeutic effect. But the level of its therapeutic effect is influenced by several factors. Our experience suggests the following points:

a) If the treatment for sprain is applied immediately after an injury occurs, then its therapeutic effect is greater, and the time required for treatment is shorter. The longer the time that elapses after an injury, the poorer the therapeutic effect and the more treatments required.

b) The effect of the treatment is related directly to the severity of the injury. This is also true in lumbar sprain. Some patients' symptoms disappear entirely after one masso-therapy session. Some are massaged as many as ten times before complete recovery is achieved. Again, when the sprain involves a partial laceration of the ligament, then the results of the treatment with masso-therapy are good. But if the ligament is completely lacerated or severed, the stability of the joint is lessened, perhaps even to the point of partial dislocation, and massage therapy will not be sufficient. In general, a surgical operation is needed, in such cases.

c) During the treatment period, proper rest should be taken. If the patient does not take proper rest, but engages in physical exercise or carries heavy loads, then the healing of the ligament will be affected.

d) An unhealed acute sprain is easily re-injured.

e) The therapeutic effect of the masso-therapy depends on the degree of skill attained by the practitioner. An uninterrupted course of treatments is also very important.

6. Bruise

Bruise is a commonly-seen injury to soft tissue. It occurs in the limbs and also in internal organs. Here we chiefly deal with the bruise of the limbs.

Etiology

Bruise is chiefly an injury to the soft tissue (including the skin, the subcutaneous tissue, the muscles, the nerves, the blood vessels, the lymphatic vessels etc.) caused by an obtuse force. At the time of injury there may occur exudations of both lymph and blood, swelling, pain and abnormality in sensation. Massage therapy treatment of this condition acts chiefly to disperse the accumulated blood and to improve the flow of vital energy and blood. It can help in exudative absorption and in improving the local nourishment of the tissues, and so is favourable to restoring the tissues to a healthy condition.

Symptoms

The local contused area immediately produces a swelling. Hemorrhage and a hematomatic mass may develop under the skin and there are sensations of pain or numbness in the swollen area. Bruises to the limbs produce differing degrees of disordered movement. A serious bruise, because of the rupture of the blood vessels and the lymphatic vessels, may produce a disturbance in the return of lymph and/or blood. Therefore it may leave a long-term swelling of the tissue and even the deposition of its exudate, together with adhesion and contracture which make the limb difficult to move.

Diagnosis

It is much easier to diagnose with a history of trauma and with local symptoms. But when the bruise is serious an x-ray examination must be made, in order to tell whether the bone is injured and to avoid mistaken diagnosis and mistaken treatment.

Treatment

In massage treatment of contusion, methods vary with the stage at which the injury is treated.

a) Contusion—acute stage:

(i) When acute symptoms are extremely obvious, place the limb in a comfortable raised position before proceeding with massage.

(ii) First, take a commonly-used acupoint near the site of the injury and apply the finger-dig and finger-vibrate methods until there is quite a strong reaction of soreness and swelling, about 1 minute.

(iii) Then, also in the area of the injury, apply the push, rub, kneading and divergent-push methods for about 2 minutes, going up and down and side to side until the accumulation dissipates and blood circulation around the site of the injury is improved.

(iv) Next, knead very lightly with the flat of the thumb or with the centre of the palm for about 1 minute at the site of the injury, kneading just lightly enough not to cause any increase in pain. Then massage around the circumference of the injury as in (iii) above for about 10–15 minutes. Finally, apply external medication in a poultice under slight pressure. For a suitable prescription, see under "Sprain of the Ankle Joint," p. 121.

b) Contusion—later stage: This refers to the period two or three days after the injury, when pain and swelling have begun to improve; or to an even later period, where swelling and impeded mobility remain.

(i) First find a commonly-used acupoint in the neighbourhood of the injured area. Then apply the finger dig and finger vibrate methods until they produce a strong reaction of soreness and a swollen feeling. This should take about 1 minute.

(ii) Use thumb or palm push methods to massage around the circumference of the injured area. In general, go from the furthest point and work in. For example on a finger or toe start from the tip of the digit. On large areas, both hands can be used. The divergent push method can be used to do both sides of the injured site. Then push and knead on the injured site, lightly. Massage on and around the injury for about 10 minutes.

(iii) If the swelling is still severe enough that pressing with a finger leaves a mark, then the finger-cut method may be applied, lightly and in a dense pattern of strokes. In the centre of the injury or where pain is evident, movements should be light and slow. Continue until there is some reduction in the swelling.

(iv) If there is adhesion, contracture and disordered mobility in a limb, apply passive manipulations such as rotation, extension or bending to help restore mobility. Be sure to avoid over-extension.

(v) In the late stages of a bruise there may be no need to apply a poultice. But a Chinese herbal fomentation may be used, as well as medical exercise and physiotherapy.

Therapeutic effect

At the acute stage of contusion, swelling and pain can be reduced immediately by massage. Generally, bruises that are not serious can be basically healed in about a week (6–7 massage sessions). Serious bruises take longer, but massage can greatly shorten the healing process here, too. At the same time it can prevent contracture, stiffening and reduced function in the joint, and lessen the contusion's residual symptoms.

Case History

Hu ———, female, age 23, student. Her left instep was run over by a horse-carriage the day before. The pain was so great that she could not walk. On examination, her left instep was seriously swollen, and there was obvious pressure-pain, but no hematomatic spot. An x-ray showed that there was no fracture and contusion was diagnosed. The methods of massage described above were applied combined with external application of Chinese herbal medication. After 4 massage sessions and three applications of herbal poultices, the swelling and pain were completely gone and she was healed.

7. Muscular Laceration

Muscle lacerations are also referred to as either "twisted" or "torn" muscles, depending on the severity of the laceration. In most cases the muscle fibre is partially torn, and complete severance of the muscle bundle is rare.

Etiology

Muscle laceration is usually produced by a sharp, uncoordinated contraction of the muscle. It can also be the result of a sudden passive or active traction. The condition is most common among athletes and those engaged in heavy labor. Muscle tissues which have already undergone pathologic changes or whose function is comparatively weak are particularly susceptible.

Symptoms

At the time of the injury, the patient is often conscious of a tearing sensation. Then contraction pain occurs in the affected group of muscles. A swollen mass forms locally due to hemorrhage under the skin. The next day, small bruised spots in the skin may appear near the injury. Over the next several days, the sharp pain at the site and the pain of the muscle contraction gradually lessen. The petechial spots are also gradually absorbed, but the swelling at the injury gradually hardens into a swollen lump, sometimes called a "knot" of extravasated blood, and this does not easily disperse. The lump causes the symptoms of motion pain and local pressure pain to persist.

Diagnosis

Diagnosis is not difficult when there are both a history of sudden, sharp injury, and the local physical signs. To ascertain whether a certain muscle or a certain group of muscles has been lacerated, do an anti-resistance test according to the site of pressure pain or swelling. The muscle that is lacerated will give a positive reaction of anti-resistance pain. With the late-stage patient one should feel the muscle for any remaining hard lump. In addition, pay special attention to whether there is the complication of muscular calcification. This occurs most often in the quadriceps muscles of the thigh and in the elbow muscles. Whenever necessary, an x-ray examination can be made.

Treatment

a) Massage: Different manipulations should be applied at different stages. If the muscular laceration is accompanied by muscular calcification then massage therapy must be temporarily delayed. However, at a later stage, when the ossification has become stable, massage may be used with caution.

(i) At the time of the injury, or within 24 hours thereafter, do not use strong, deep massage. Lightly and slowly apply the palm rub method, starting at the circumference and moving gradually to the center of the injury. Do not continue for too long. Immediately after massage, a medication for trauma is externally applied and bound around the wounded area under some pressure (see opposite).

(ii) After two or three days, hemorrhage will have ceased, and swelling and small bruised spots in the skin will appear. Then the flat palm push method is applied above and below the injured area, pushing from the distal point toward the proximal. This process is repeated about ten times. Then the base and the edge of the palm are employed for light kneading of the swollen area, going from the circumference to the center of the injury and then from the center to the circumference. Do not use enough force to cause pain. To the superficial bruises around the injury, apply the finger-cut method. After massaging, apply a trauma medication (see opposite) and bind the wound, or use a medication for reducing pain and swelling (see p. 121).

(iii) If a hard swollen knot and motion pain remain in the late stage of the injury, but the complication of muscular calcification is not diagnosed, deep kneading can be applied locally, or the flat-thumb push or thumb-tip push method can be used. Then, while the push and kneading methods are being applied, add passive manipulations such as the rotation and stretch methods. Rotate and knead at the same time, with the amount of rotation or stretching not great enough to cause pain. Conclude with the shake method.

b) *Other treatment:* Rest must be taken at the acute stage of a muscle laceration. External application of medication, under pressure, is extremely important. Various physical therapies can be used, in combination with medical exercise.

Therapeutic Effect

Massage applied to the muscle laceration at an early stage must be light. Massage applied to a case in its late stages has the effect of reducing the swelling, eliminating the superficial bruises, loosening the tendons and ligaments, killing pain and restoring mobility.

Medication for Trauma

The following ten herbs are reduced to a fine powder, mixed with syrup to form a paste and applied externally to the wound.

Huangbo	1 liang	Phellodendron chinense Schneid. (bark)
Xuejie	1 liang	Daemonorops draco Bl. (dragon's blood)
Dahuang	2 liang	Rheum officinale Baill. (root stem)
Mutong	1 qian	Akebia trifoliata (Thunb.) Koidz (fruit)
Yanhusuo	2 qian	Corydalis yanhusuo (rhizome)
Qianghuo	5 qian	Notopterygium incisum Ting. (root)
Duhuo	5 qian	Angelica pubescens Maxim. (root)
Baizhi	5 qian	Angelica anomala (root)
Muxiang	5 qian	Saussurea lappa Clarke (costusroot)
Xixin	5 qian	Asarum sieboldi Mig. (root)

Case History

Sha ———, female, age 19, high-school student. Right after participating in sports she felt a sudden pain in the inner side of the left thigh. This had continued for two weeks. The pain became sharper, at the inner side of the thigh near the groin, after she ran a race. On examination, there were pressure pains in the adductor muscle of the left thigh and at the attachment of the pelvic area. The muscle was quite tense. Abductor resistance test positive. Laceration of the adductor muscle of the left thigh was diagnosed. After massage was applied as above four times, the aching, motion pain and local pressure-pain were all gone. She was told to rest for a week before participating in sports again. Upon visiting her a month later we found that she had completely recovered her athletic ability.

8. Fractures of the Limbs

In Chinese medical books on the treatment of wounds, eight massage therapy methods for setting fractures are mentioned: the feel, connect, correct, raise, press, rub, push and grasp methods. The four former methods are mainly concerned with setting the bone and the latter four are mainly concerned with massage. But setting the bone is combined with massage, and in massage it is sometimes necessary to pay attention to setting the bone. The aim in setting a bone is to restore the fractured bone to its proper position. The purpose of massage is to remove swelling, to disperse extravasated blood, to accelerate the circulation of the blood, to relieve adhesion, and to prevent articular dysfunction. These are the two inseparable parts of the set of methods for treating fractures. Moreover, they reflect the union of movement and stillness in the methods used by Chinese medical science for the treatment of fractures.

The purpose of reduction is to restore function. But if in treatment one pays attention only to reduction, then even though the fracture can be brought into proper alignment, the function of the limb may still be impeded, and the final goal of treatment not reached. Therefore, massage must be used during the whole course of fracture reduction. During the period when the position of the fractured bone needs frequent correction, frequent massage is also advisable.

There are already many specialized books on fracture reduction, so here we will not go into great detail. The functional disturbances that arise from fractures, and the problems of how to use massage under the differing conditions of various fractures, are introduced below.

Etiology

After a bone has been fractured, various degrees of disturbance of function can develop. The most important factors in this are described below. We analyze these factors to coincide with the massage techniques that are effective in preventing disordered functions.

a) A fracture that cannot be reduced or that is poorly realigned can leave such malformations as angle-formation, malposition and shortening that affect the function of the limb.

b) The muscles and ligaments attached to the fractured bone lose their tension after fracture, producing spasm, scarring and calcification, and affecting the function of the limb.

c) There is much hemorrhage and exudation in the soft tissues surrounding a closed fracture. Some fractures must be reduced by surgical operation, and much hemorrhage and exudation can also result from the operation. The hemorrhage and exuded materials form fibrin depositions, or the hematoma becomes fibrosed giving rise to adhesions and ankylosis of the fractured area and of the surrounding joints, and affecting function. All the above effects are much greater in an open fracture.

d) Because of long-term immobilization of a fractured limb, free circulation of blood in the limb is reduced. This can promote fibrin deposition. At the same time, long immobilization can cause adhesion in the synovial membrane of a joint and atrophy and contracture of the muscles, resulting in reduced function.

e) Fractures that involve injury to the nerves and blood-vessels can also result in disordered function.

Symptoms

Since the site of the fracture and the extent of the wound differ from case to case, so the symptoms manifested differ as well. The main symptoms that follow a fracture are pain, obvious local swelling, deformation and disordered function. In open fractures, there is an open wound in the soft tissue. If there is injury to nerves and blood-vessels, phenomena such as hemorrhage and paralysis are likely to be present.

Diagnosis

Based on the symptoms and external signs, use the hand to meticulously examine the injury. Generally, a preliminary diagnosis can be made as to whether or not there is fracture or malposition. When no x-ray examination is available, this is the chief method of diagnosis. An x-ray examination is necessary for definite diagnosis of fracture and of specific phenomena associated with certain fractures. For disordered function, a protractor is used to measure the amount of movement in the joint; the circumference of a limb can be measured with a linen tape to ascertain the amount of swelling and muscular atrophy. At the same time, muscle contraction and muscle tension can be measured with a grasp-strength meter or a pull-strength meter[1] to estimate the strength of the muscles.

_____

1. "pull-strength meter" refers to a pulley.

Treatment

a) *Massage:* Immediately after the injury:

(i) Following a fracture, manipulation is used to set the fractured bone back into its proper position and it is immobilized with a small splint. When the immobilizing splint is opened up to change the poultice, massage can be applied to the fracture site and to the whole wounded limb. In the massage, the practitioner's sense of touch contributes to the proper alignment of the broken bone. If necessary, a further alignment can be made. Traction therapy is adopted for the treatment of some types of fracture. After traction, massage can also be applied to the fracture site and the wounded limb. When reduction and immobilization of the fractured bone are not required, massage can be applied to the fractured bone and the wounded limb right after the fracture occurs. After surgical reduction of a fracture or in open fracture, massage can be applied to the circumference of the incision and to the whole injured limb. In a small number of cases, a plaster cast is used for immobilization, and massage can be applied only to the parts of the limb not included in the cast.

(ii) Massage is carried out in a sitting position for fractured upper limbs, but for fractured lower limbs only a lying position can be used. For limbs that are immobilized or in traction, apply massage with the patient in any comfortable position.

(iii) At this stage, the most important methods of massage are the palm push and palm rub methods, or the light kneading and light pinch methods. Usually, one pushes from the far end of the limb toward the body. A light massage is applied in the area of the fracture, but a somewhat heavier one can be applied to areas further away. Apply passive manipulations such as the extension, bending, and rotation methods to joints at some distance from the site of the fracture. On the upper part of the fractured limb, select some commonly-used acupoints and apply the finger dig, thumb push, and finger vibrate methods. Finally the push and rub methods are again performed. Massage for about 15 minutes each time.

After the fracture has healed:

(i) The kneading and pinch methods should be applied to the fracture and the whole wounded limb. Massage with one or both hands, and go from the distal to the proximal point. The rub-roll method is used for the upper limbs and the roll method is used for lower limbs. Sometimes the palm vibrate, light hammer and light pat methods can be used so that the effects of the massage penetrate deeply into the muscles.

(ii) Passive manipulations such as extension, bending, rotation and shaking should be applied to the injured limb in appropriate amounts. When performing these manipulations, special attention must be paid to whether or not movement is possible in the joints of the injured limb. The manipulations must be vigorous, but dexterous rather than rough and violent. Nevertheless, some progress in the mobility of the wounded limb should be made at each treatment.

b) Other treatment: Treatment with Chinese herbal medicines can be combined with the other treatment of a newly-fractured bone. After the fracture has healed, in addition to massage, the use of medical exercise should be emphasized. Differing exercise programs must be drawn up to focus on different sites of injury and differing requirements for restoration of disordered function. These programs should consist mainly of exercises that emphasize development of muscle strength and articular mobility. Exercises involving lifting sandbags are very effective in developing muscle strength (see p 108).

Therapeutic Effect

Massage therapy is very important in the prevention and cure of post-fracture disordered function. In general the earlier it is applied, the less will function remain disordered. Even if disordered function has already appeared, massage therapy and medical exercise should still be used. If the proper techniques are selected, then the patient will have the confidence to persevere in carrying out the exercise program, and mobility can usually be restored. In the few cases where deformed structures cannot be restored to their original state, crippling can be reduced to a minimum if the patient is determined to resolutely carry out the program of medical exercise, thereby developing his latent compensatory abilities.

Case History No. 1

Feng ———, female, age 54, poor peasant. Had been injured two hours earlier, when she fell and used the carpal part of her right hand to break her fall. Examination revealed evident swelling of the wrist, which was deformed into a fork shape. By manual examination we found that there was a fracture at the end of the radius near the wrist. The end fragment had moved backwards in relation to the radius. Fracture of the distal end of the radius was diagnosed (Colles fracture). With two people applying traction, the correct and raise methods were used to bring the fractured bones back into proper position. A poultice of *Jinhuang San*[1] was applied. The back of the forearm and the side of the palm were immobilized with a small splint.

When the dressing was changed on the third day, the swelling was still evident. Examination revealed that the alignment of the fractured bones was quite good and that they had not moved. After massaging the fractured area and again immobilizing and binding it up, massage was applied every day to the part of the hand not covered by the splint, and the patient was told to exercise it herself. On the seventh day the swelling was already obviously reduced. External application of medication was stopped. The wrist was simply bound up with a dressing and kept in a small splint, which was removed once a day for massage and passive manipulation.

After three weeks, there was no local pain, the swelling had almost completely disappeared and there was no disturbance of function in the wrist or in the forearm. The splint was removed and all treatment was stopped. The patient was told to continue a program of exercise and massage, and to do light practical work such as twisting cotton into threads.

Case History No. 2

Fan ———, male, age 49, worker. His fracture of the upper third of the ulna was placed in a cast for two months. When the fracture healed and the cast was taken off there was disordered function in the elbow and in the shoulder,

---

1. "Golden Powder," a Chinese herbal mixture for external use.

particularly the elbow. It extended to only 14 degrees and bent to only 86 degrees, so that the scope of its mobility was only 54 degrees. The muscles of the right arm had atrophied to the point that grasp-strength was zero.

After ten applications of the aforementioned massage, in combination with medical exercise, the mobility of the shoulder had returned to normal. The mobility of the elbow was also largely restored: it extended to 172 degrees and bent to 50 degrees, giving a range of mobility of 122 degrees. The grasp-strength of the muscles had already reached 15 kilograms, enough to permit normal life and work. The treatment was stopped and the patient was told to persist in a program of medical exercise.

9. Impairment of the Genu-Meniscus

When external forces to which the knee cannot adapt, such as twisting, stretching, squeezing or pressing, are imposed upon it, the meniscus cartilage may be torn. Depending on the location and extent of the tear, the fissure may be longitudinal or transverse; it may be in the middle of the genu meniscus in the front angle, in the rear angle, or in the edge. It can be large and deep or only a small transverse tear. The direction of the twisting, the amount to which the knee is bent at the time of the injury and the amount of force involved all make for variations in the fissure that is formed.

Symptoms

(i) Pain and a sound in the knee: After the knee joint undergoes an injury there is often pain and a sound in the joint, usually accompanied by swelling. The swelling goes down spontaneously after a short time, but the pain and the sound usually remain. The pain is sharp and often is produced when the knee is extended to a certain point. The sound is produced at the same time, although there are some patients who themselves cannot hear it. Because of unusual sound and pain in the knee, normal life and work are usually affected.

(ii) Locking and unlocking symptom: The patient often complains that something suddenly gets caught in the knee joint, impeding its bend-extend movement, but says that after rubbing or lightly swinging the knee, the joint frees itself. When the locking symptom occurs, the newly-injured patient often has swelling in the knee joint. In old injuries, locking of the joint is often no longer accompanied by swelling. Some other conditions show symptoms similar to this locking, and these should be discriminated. Cases with typical locking and unlocking symptoms usually involve quite severe tears.

(iii) Asthenia and atrophy in the leg: After the knee joint is injured there is generally adynamia in the leg, and atrophy of the thigh muscle.

Diagnosis

Injuries of the knee joint are quite complicated and diagnosis is rather difficult. Apart from looking at etiology and symptoms, three other types of examination should be made:

(i) Pressure pain: Search out a fixed pressure pain on the injured side of the intra-articular space. The site of the pressure-pain will aid in diagnosing whether the injury is in the front, middle, or rear of the cartilage.

(ii) Have the patient lie supine. The examiner supports the affected knee with one hand and with the other hand holds the foot of the affected leg. Then rotate the calf inward and outward, while at the same time bending and extending the knee. Rotate outward to check the medial meniscus, rotate inward to check the lateral meniscus. Pain and sound, or the feeling of a sound in the examiner's hand, will be produced at a different angle of extension of the knee, depending on the site of the fissure.

(iii) If necessary, the diagnosis can be made more accurate by x-ray examination.

Treatment

a) *Massage*: (i) The patient lies prone. Massage by the kneading and roll methods is applied to the muscles of the calf and the thigh on the affected side, going up and down the leg several times.

(ii) The patient then switches to a supine position. Massage by the roll and pinch methods is applied to the anterior thigh muscles of the affected side, going up and down several times.

(iii) With the flat-thumb push method, first massage the *xiyan* "eye of the knee" acupoints on either side of the patella. Then massage along both sides of the articular space, going backward as far as the popliteal fossa. Go back and forth along each side several times.

(iv) Dip the fingertips in medicinal liquor (see p. 78) and apply the kneading and rub methods on and around the point of the pressure-pain, gradually using greater force. When the medicinal liquor dries, dip again and repeat, in all about 8–10 times, until a feeling of warmth arises in the area.

(v) Finally the light pat, kneading, and rub methods can be applied to the calf and thigh of the affected side of the leg.

b) Other Treatment: Twice daily massage can be combined with applications of a fomentation of Chinese herbs and with medical exercise. At night, dress the affected side with a Chinese herbal preparation for moving the vital energy and enlivening the blood (see p.121).

Therapeutic Effect

Massage often has no effect on a serious tear of the meniscus or on the loose bodies of the knee joint. But it usually has a satisfactory therapeutic effect on small or marginal fissures. Generally, subjective symptoms and even objective physical signs can be made to disappear by means of massage, and the ability to work and athletic ability can be restored to normal. However, the course of treatment is quite long, usually 1–3 months.

Case History

Liu ——, male, age 22, soccer player. His right knee had already been painful for over two months. In a football match, he had used his right leg in a challenge for the ball, but his opponent had suddenly stepped on the outside of Liu's right knee, causing him to fall backward. He felt a sharp pain in the knee, which immediately became swollen. It became better after a few days' rest, but there continued to be pain and a sound in the medial right knee when he moved it. Sometimes it locked, but he could unlock it by moving it a bit.

On examination there was a pressure pain under the kneecap near the medial accessory ligament of the right knee. When the right knee rotated outward to about 140 degrees, there was pain and a sound. An anterior-site fissure in the medial semilunar fibrocartilage of the right knee was clinically diagnosed. The total course of treatment with the above-mentioned massage and fomentation of Chinese herbal medicine lasted 56 days. By then the subjective symptoms had completely vanished, and examination revealed neither pain nor sound. Since the knee was completely healed, treatment was stopped.

10. Patello-malacia

Etiology

Softening of the kneecap (patello-malacia) is also called "patellar strain." The articular surface of the knee, particularly the articular surface of the knee-cap, suffers from long-term and excessive incorrect movement, so that a straining injury develops. This is a common type of sports injury.

It is generally thought that the kneecap has the function of increasing the strength of the quadriceps thigh muscle. But when the knee is extended to about 150 degrees, not only is the strength of the quadriceps femoris-kneecap structure at its greatest, but the kneecap is facing a compression force of the articular surface with the femur, which is also at its greatest. Therefore, making too many forceful movements from a half-crouching position, or doing too many of such things as getting up from a crouch with a heavy weight, or running backwards, can cause the cartilage of the articular surface of the knee cap to develop a series of degenerative pathological changes that result in this condition.

In addition, in our clinical work we have come to understand that other composite injuries around the knee joint usually occur in the patient with patellar strain. A relation of cause and effect may exist between these injuries and the patellar strain.

Symptoms

Generally, the development of the disease is gradual. At the onset the patient complains of discomfort in the knee, or a feeling of weakness. When it becomes more severe there is a scraping pain under the patella, which disappears after a period of movement. The pain becomes more intense after rest, even causing lameness. When it reaches the severe stage, walking can give pain, going up and down staircases can make it worse, and crouching is impossible.

Diagnosis

A preliminary diagnosis can be made on the basis of etiology and symptoms, but three further types of examination should also be made as follows:

(i) *Kneecap press test:* Have the knee extended straight. With the surface of the palm press directly on the knee cap. In more serious cases, there may be an immediate painful reaction. The amount of force required and the painfulness of the reaction serve to determine the degree of positive reaction.

(ii) *Finger-press test:* With the knee extended straight, tell the patient to relax the quadriceps muscle of the thigh. Then the examiner with one hand pushes the kneecap inward and outward. With the fingertips of his other hand, he presses under the kneecap; this often produces a painful reaction. Note whether the pain is on the inside or the outside of the knee, and describe its degree.

(iii) *The kneecap rub test:* With the palm of the hand press against the kneecap and slide it with a rubbing motion toward the inside and then the outside of the knee. Do not use too much force. At this time the patient will feel a painful scraping sensation, and the examiner may also be conscious of a scraping feeling from the kneecap surface. Both the site and the extent of the scraping sensation can be described.

Treatment

a) *Massage*: (i) Using the prone position, a massage by means of the roll or the pinch method is applied on both the thigh and the calf areas. Use enough force to work deep into the muscles. Go up and down the leg several times.

(ii) A supine position is taken. The above methods are again applied on both the thigh and the calf areas, and the thumb-push method can be applied to the muscle-group of the calf and the front of the tibia.

(iii) Bend the patient's knee slightly and support the knee with a pillow. Do a thumb-tip push and a flat-thumb push on both sides of the space below the kneecap and on the subpatellar ligament area. Then the push method is applied around the circumference of the knee. Finally, do more pushing against the bursa above the kneecap.

(iv) With the tips of the five fingers, grasp the outer and inner margins of the kneecap. Then, using finger-force, apply a rubbing motion all around the edge of the kneecap. Do everything possible to avoid causing pain by sliding the kneecap from side to side. Then techniques such as the finger dig and finger-vibrate are applied to acupoints in the area such as *zusanli*, *xuehai*, *yinling-quan* and *yanglingquan*.

(v) Finally again apply the kneading and rub methods to the thigh and the calf. The entire massage of the leg should take about 15 minutes.

(*b*) *Other Treatment*: To raise the therapeutic effect to a higher level, massage can be combined with fomentations, physical therapy, etc. During the course of treatment, rest or partial rest must be emphasized so as to prevent wasting atrophies from developing, and a suitable program of medical exercise must be prescribed (see Diagram 71, p. 109).

Massage in treatment of this disease is only part of the total treatment, and hence its therapeutic effect must be judged as part of the therapeutic effect of the treatment as a whole. But the patient does generally report that after each massage session he immediately feels relaxation and comfort in the knees, thigh, and calf areas.

Case History

Chou ——, male, age 20, wrestler. His right knee had gradually become more painful over the past three months. When he crouched down the pain became worse, and this affected his training. Examination: Patellar-press and patellar-rub tests on the knee were both positive. A finger-press test found pressure pain beneath both edges of the patella. Strain of the patella of the right knee was diagnosed. The aforementioned methods of massage were used in combination with fomentations of Chinese medicinal herbs. After ten treatments, the painful symptoms and the physical signs were completely gone, and he had recovered.

11. Flatfoot and Foot Strain

Etiology

This condition occurs mainly among workers who stand too much, or who work half-crouching, and among athletes, especially teenagers. Thus it may be called an occupational or athletic strain. The condition usually develops because the tissue-structures in the area have not yet solidified, while body-weight has developed more quickly, and the load placed on calf and foot in labour or sports exceeds the ability of the structures in the area to support it.

Strain of the foot area is very often occompanied by secondary sagging of the arch of the foot. This is because the body weight is too great, and the muscles and ligaments of the calf and foot that maintain the arch cannot support the load. As the muscles that maintain the arch, such as the anterior and posterior tibial muscles and the peroneus longus and brevis muscles, lose tension because of over-exhaustion, the force of the body weight is all imposed upon the ligaments that support the arch. The ligaments are gradually pulled slack, resulting in the arched bone structure of the foot being unable to maintain itself, and the arch sags. Over a long period of time, this leads to strain and to a deformation that is not easily reversed.

Symptoms

At the onset there may only be symptoms such as weakness of the affected foot, easy tiring and inability to walk very far. In the early stages, there is the symptom of pain, usually pain in the sole, but sometimes a spasmodic pain in the gastrocnemius, or radiating pain in a certain muscle group. During examination, a pressure pain in a certain muscle group can often be found, too, and occasionally resistance pain can be discovered in the same muscle group. Generally, there is excessive tension in the muscles, and also tension and a pressure pain in the deep tissues and ligaments of the sole of the foot, as well as a mild limp.

In the late stage a slight club foot tendency appears. At that time the pain usually lessens. Generally the arch of the foot gradually becomes flatter, particularly as the scaphoid bone gradually collapses. In the knotted area of the scaphoid bone an obvious pressure pain appears, affecting labour and sports.

Diagnosis

In the early stage, diagnosis is easier and can be based on the symptoms and a local examination. At a later stage, an x-ray of the foot area should be taken. Apart from the changes in the bones that are characteristic of flatfoot, sometimes such complications as stress periostitis or lacerated fracture can be found at some muscle attachments. Or else symptoms that ensue from collapse of the arch can be seen, such as strain induced arthritis of the small bones of the feet.

Treatment

a) *Massage:* (i) First have the patient lie face down. The shin is supported with a pillow so that the leg rests comfortably. Apply the flat-thumb push method or the roll method from the back of the knee space downward; use the thumb push method on the popliteal space and on both sides of the Achilles tendon; and use the roll method on the gastrocnemius (or calf) muscle. Go back and forth several times. Apply the finger-dig and thumb kneading methods to acupoints such as *weizhong, chengshan, taixi* and *kunlun.*

(ii) Then have the patient turn over onto his or her back. Massage using the thumb push method or the roll method, going back and forth several times over the extensor muscle in front of the tibia, as far as the instep area. At the same time apply massage to acupoints such as *zusanli, yanglingquan* and *jiexi.*

(iii) With one hand, firmly grasp the bottom of the patient's foot, and apply the pinch method to the instep of the foot. Start by pinching a wide area, then pinch along between each of the metatarsal bones. Finally, do a deep pinching along the flexor and extensor muscles of the calf and the muscle bundles of the peroneus longus and brevis. This should be done for about 5–10 minutes.

(iv) Have the patient actively or passively shake his ankle. Then apply the rub-roll and the vibrate methods on the calf and the foot area to conclude the massage.

b) *Other treatment*: In the early stages of calf and foot strain, fomentations of or soaking in Chinese herbal medicines for relaxing the muscles and improving circulation of the blood can be used. At a later stage, if the arch has not already fallen, a corrective padding in the shoe can be used as well. At the same time have the patient do medical exercises to strengthen the muscles of the calf and the foot. In the course of treatment, attention should be paid to resting the affected area.

Therapeutic Effect

In early cases, the symptoms improve markedly after one massage session and are completely cured after several sessions. At a later stage, after the secondary strain of flatfoot has already appeared, results are poorer and the course of treatment required is longer. But in general symptoms such as pain, etc., can be gotten rid of, malformation can be improved, and athletic ability can be restored.

Case History No. 1

Liu ———, male, age 20, foundry-worker. He was a demobilized soldier who had worked in a foundry for only two months. Because he worked in a crouch for long periods at a time, an aching had developed in the gastrocnemius muscles of both calves. The pain had been getting worse for the past several days. He could no longer crouch down, was unable to stand for long, and had a limp. Examination: There was tension and pressure pain in the gastrocnemius muscles of both legs. Slight backward bending of the ankle gave unbearable pain. The diagnosis was occupational strain of the gastrocnemius muscle.

After one massage treatment the painful symptoms were immediately mitigated, the muscles relaxed and the pressure pain abated. The ankle could be actively bent backward about 80 degrees and his limp was obviously improved. After one more massage treatment on the following day, the symptoms disappeared, and treatment was stopped.

Case History No. 2

Zhou ———, male, age 24, cadre. The patient's work was mainly out-of-doors and required him to do quite a bit of walking. For more than a month, because he had been walking too much, he had felt pain in both feet, especially in the left foot. The pain was a swelling pain that extended up to the calf, causing him to limp. Examination: Both feet were slightly flat and there was slight swelling in the instep of the left foot. There were mild pressure pains along the medial margins of the arches of both feet, in the condyli laterales and in the Achilles tendons. After only three treatments by the methods of massage outlined above, the swelling gradually dissipated and the pain went away. He walked normally again, so treatment was stopped.

12. Shoulder Periarthritis

Shoulder periarthritis is also called "frozen shoulder," or "congealed shoulder". It is common among middle-aged and older people, and therefore is called "fifty-year-old's shoulder," as well. It usually develops on only one side.

Etiology

This condition consists essentially of inflammatory changes in the soft tissues around the shoulder joint. The cause of it is not yet completely understood. Certain cases may be related to trauma or chronic strain. Doctors of Chinese medicine consider it to be caused by wind, cold and moisture attacking a shoulder that is vulnerable due to the weakness of old age, deficiencies of blood and vital energy, and nutritional imbalance. Today there are those who consider it a "collagen disease."

Symptoms

For no apparent reason, soreness, weakness, and impeded mobility gradually develop in the shoulder area. At the onset of the disease, pain is usually the main symptom. Soreness spreads through the shoulder area, and is often particularly noticeable at the front of the shoulder. It sometimes radiates into the forearm. Raising the arm from the side and rotating it outward increases the pain, so the affected shoulder is usually held in a fixed position. At the same time, the patient often feels weak, or unable to continue for very long, when he does things like carrying something on his shoulder.

When a later stage is reached, the aching symptoms are often gradually reduced, but the mobility of the shoulder joint is increasingly impeded. Especially difficult are abduction and outward rotation; adduction and forward flexing are also somewhat impeded. Therefore, not only is productive labor affected, but movements involved in writing, eating, combing the hair, and putting clothes on also become difficult. Whenever there is wet weather the local symptoms become more severe.

Diagnosis

Diagnosis based on history and symptoms is quite easy. Examine the external appearance of the shoulder. Generally there will be muscular atrophy in the shoulder area. Periarthritis must be distinguished from acute injuries such as fracture and dislocation. At the same time examine the shoulder area for any specific pressure pain in the shoulder, note the site of any motion-pain in the forearm, and measure the amount of movement in the shoulder. These observations will make it possible to apply the correct treatment.

Treatment

a) Massage: General method and sequence:

(i) Have the patient take a sitting position, with his shoulders relaxed. First the thumb-rub and the flat-thumb push methods are applied on the back and scapula areas of both shoulders. Then with the base of the palm apply the kneading and rub methods or the roll method to the scapulo-dorsal area of the affected shoulder. Go from light to heavy and shallow to deep, massaging for about 5-10 minutes, until the local area feels comfortable and warm, and the muscles are relaxed and soft.

(ii) Slowly and dexterously apply the pinch method. You can go from the shoulder down to the upper arm, concentrating on the front of the shoulder. Repeat several times. Combine this with massage of such acupoints as *fengchi, jianjing, jianliao, jianyu, jianzhen* and *hegu*, using the finger dig and finger vibrate methods or the thumb tip push method.

(iii) Then the light hammer method or the light pat method is applied on the shoulder area. At the same time the shake and rotation methods are also used. The range of the shaking and rotation should gradually be increased.

(iv) Finally knead and rub the shoulder, neck, upper back, and arm on the affected side, and finish with a rub-roll massage of the arm.

Methods for specific situations:

(i) When the case is in its early stages, where pain is evident and the patient is weak, one should make more use of the push and roll methods, or else apply conduction oil or medicinal liquor and use the chafe method. Make less use of the shake and rotation methods. If slight rotation immediately gives rise to severe pain, then do not use the rotation method at all for a while.

(ii) With a case in its later stages, when impeded mobility is the main symptom, and the patient's general condition is comparatively good, make moving the joint the main treatment. Do a passive movement of the shoulder with one hand, while with the other hand applying the knead, rub, and roll methods to the shoulder area, particularly any specific painful site. See Diagrams 74 and 75. Attention must be paid to gradually enlarging the range of movement. When the movement of the shoulder joint has been reasonably well restored, stretching of the limb should be combined with the other aspects of the treatment.

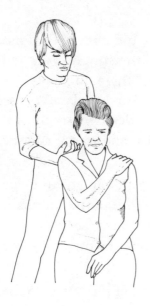

DIAGRAM 74

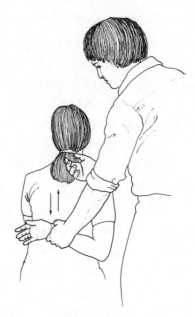

DIAGRAM 75

(iii) In cases of long-term illness, particularly when movement disturbance is comparatively severe and restoration of mobility is not evident, the extend method and the grasp method may also be used on the shoulder. In some such

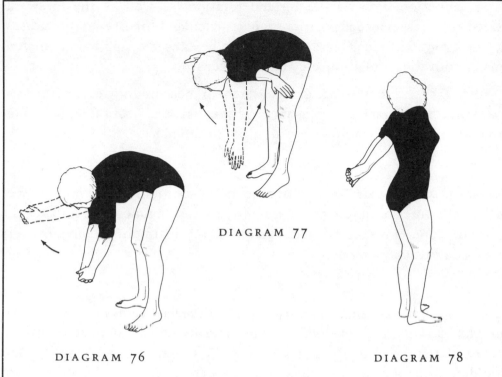

DIAGRAM 77

DIAGRAM 76   DIAGRAM 78

Medical Exercise

(i) *Shoulder lift:* Bend forward at the waist, let the arms hang down and clasp the hands. Swing the arms forward, gradually increasing the distance that they swing. See Diagram 76.

(ii) *Shoulder abduction:* Bend at the waist and let the upper limbs hang down. Swing them naturally left and right, gradually increasing the range of motion. See Diagram 77.

(iii) *Shoulder back-extension:* Stand with feet shoulder-width apart and hands clasped palm-outward behind the back. Use the sound hand to stretch the affected hand as far out backwards as possible without bending the body forward. See Diagram 78.

(iv) *Shoulder circles:* Stand with feet set shoulder-width apart and the arms held out straight to each side. Move the arms round and round, first forward and then backward, gradually increasing the size of the circles formed.

cases, abduction, forward flexing and rotation, as well as the foreward-rotated and back-extended positions, give particular difficulty. In these cases, the energy-system pluck method can often be effective, applied at the tendons of both the deltoid muscle and the biceps.

b) *Other Treatment*: Massage can be the main measure for treating this disease, but other therapies such as medical exercise, physical therapy, and internal administration of drugs are all quite beneficial.

Therapeutic Effect

Massage is quite satisfactory for treating this condition. It not only relieves pain, but restores or improves the mobility of the shoulder, and restores the ability to work. However, the period required for treatment is comparatively long, usually about a month.

Case History

Wang ——, male, age 49, schoolteacher. Over the past eight months, his left shoulder had gradually developed soreness and disturbed mobility. He had no history of trauma. Examination: No specific external changes in the left shoulder. Mild muscular atrophy of the upper arm. Left shoulder abducted to 40 degrees. The pain became more severe when the shoulder was rotated outward. Forward bending and backward extension also restricted. There were pressure pains in the middle and front parts of the shoulder. Shoulder periarthritis was diagnosed.

After 39 treatments by the methods of massage mentioned above, in combination with medical exercise, the soreness gradually vanished. The range of the shoulder's movement was restored to normal, with abduction to 90 degrees. He could do his normal work and treatment was stopped. Upon visiting him some time later we found that there had been no recurrence.

13. Tenovaginitis

Tenovaginitis is a condition involving chronic traumatic inflammation of a tendon sheath. It is seen most often as tenovaginitis of the short extensor muscle and long abductor muscles of the thumb. This is also called "constricting tenovaginitis." Here we will deal only with tenovaginitis at this site, taking it as an example. It is introduced below. The treatment for other tenovaginitises, such as that of the foot, is similar.

Etiology

This condition is caused by prolonged abrasion. Therefore, activities that require sustained abduction of the thumb, such as washing clothes, carrying children, and athletic activities, all tend to bring it on. In addition, the short extensor muscles and long abductor muscles both pass through the tendon groove in the radial styloid process area. Since the bottom of the tendon sulcus is uneven, the tendons of the two muscles are constricted within a relatively hard, narrow sheath. When they are in motion, they can easily scrape against one another, thereby giving rise to tenovaginitis.

Symptoms

The patient feels pain in the base of the thumb, on the outside of the radial styloid process and elsewhere. There is also slight swelling and there may be a feeling of constriction and pressure-pain. When the thumb is adducted into a fist and the wrist slants toward the ulnar side, intense pain is felt at the radial styloid process. When the condition is severe, the thumb becomes fixed in the outstretched position. This is because the wall of the tendon-sheath grows thick and constricted. A hard mass can be discovered by local palpation.

Diagnosis

Diagnosis is easy, based on etiology and symptoms. However, cases should be distinguished as to whether they are at an early or a late stage.

Treatment

a) *Massage:* (i) The patient takes either a sitting position, or a supine one. The forearm is supported by a pillow. First the palm-heel kneading method is applied on the back of the hand and of the forearm. Then continue with the roll method, going up and down several times.

(ii) Rotate the forearm and the hand backward so that the radial side faces upward. Again the roll method is applied starting from the thumb area and going up as far as the elbow area. At first, pain may occur as you pass over the radial styloid process, so light pressure may be used. After a while, when pain is no longer felt at the radial styloid process, the force of the massage may gradually be increased. Next the pinch method is applied to the extensor-muscle area of the whole forearm.

(iii) The therapist grasps the affected hand with one of his hands, firmly pressing down on the affected thumb. With his other hand, he applies the roll method of massage up and down the affected tendon sheaths. While massaging, move the affected hand backward and forward and from side to side. At this time, the patient will probably feel some pain, so the amount of force used must be adjusted.

b) *Other Treatments*: A fomentation or bath of Chinese herbs may be used at the same time as the massage. During the treatment period, the affected part should be rested. With cases in their later stages, if massage cannot ease the stenotic symptoms, then surgical treatment should be adopted.

Therapeutic Effect

In early-stage cases, several massage treatments can eliminate the symptoms. In late stage cases, the course of treatment is generally rather long, but the stenosis can gradually be relieved, and the symptoms eliminated.

Case History

Ge ——, male, age 57, bricklayer. The radial side of his right forearm had been painful for three days. As a result he could neither pick up nor lay bricks. Examination: There were both a slight swelling and an obvious pressure pain in the radial styloid process of the right hand. He could not open or close his thumb. The local pain became severe when the thumb was bent toward the center of the palm. Traumatic tenovaginitis in the short extensor and long abductor muscles of the thumb of the right hand was diagnosed. After the above methods of massage for tenovaginitis had been applied seven times, the local swelling and pain were completely eliminated. He resumed work as usual, and treatment ceased.

14. Torticollis (Wryneck)

In China torticollis is called "falling off the pillow," "lost neck," or "lost pillow." This neck condition is noticed on waking when a sudden pain is felt and the head cannot be freely turned. Torticollis occurs also as a result of trauma. A minor case may last a few days and clear up spontaneously. A severe case may last for a long time, and the pain may become increasingly severe. The therapeutic effects of massage therapy on torticollis are quite good.

Etiology

Torticollis occurs either when one is extremely tired and sleeping exposed to draught giving rise to muscle-spasms or myo-fasciitis; or else when the synovial membrane of one of the small joints of the cervical vertebrae becomes inlaid, or there is a partial dislocation.

Symptoms

There is a severe pain in the neck that becomes worse when the neck is turned. These symptoms usually manifest themselves suddenly, after awakening from a sound sleep. This is the typical wryneck. The symptoms may also occur after a wrenching or twisting movement of the neck or under conditions where the head is held in a fixed position, while the body suddenly leans forward. However, the pain in the neck may occur suddenly without any of these histories. Sometimes there is just a pulling sensation in the neck, and the symptoms set in gradually, recurring often and becoming worse, especially when the neck is exposed to cold.

Diagnosis

This condition is not difficult to diagnose by pathogenic history and typical symptoms. The stiffness in the neck can be discovered by local examination. There will be neither redness, nor swelling, but there will be limitation of movement in bending, extending, and rotating the head. There is often a pressure pain on the lower side of the back of the head (corresponding to portions of the sternocleidomastoid muscle and of the trapezius). Wryneck is usually caused by a muscular spasm, or inflammation, but cases in which there is a pressure pain at a small joint of the cervical vertebrae usually result from synovial inlay.

Treatment

a) Massage: Normal methods and sequence— (i) The patient is seated, while the practitioner stands behind him and to one side. First, the flat-thumb push method is applied to the shoulders and the upper back, especially on the affected side. This will make the patient more comfortable and relaxed.

(ii) With the thumb and index finger continue by applying the knead and grasp massages to the muscle group at the back of the neck, starting from the *fengchi* acupoint down along the muscles and around to the *jianjing* acupoint on the affected side, grasping the acupoint 2–3 times, until the vital energy appears. In this manner knead and grasp repeatedly, until relaxation of the muscle group in the patient's neck area is achieved.

(iii) Apply the neck-rotation method. (See Diagram 38, p. 41.) Be quite certain to avoid producing any pain. The range of movement should be small. While you are turning his neck, ask the patient to relax his neck muscles. Wait till the neck muscles are completely relaxed, and no resistance to the rotation remains. Then sharply twist the neck. Finally, again knead and grasp the muscle group at the back of the neck 2–3 times.

Special Procedures

(i) When a semi-dislocated joint is suspected, the neck-rotation method is not advisable. After relaxation of the neck area by the normal massage, a neck-lifting manipulation can be used: Ask the patient to sit cross-legged on the ground. The practitioner stands behind the patient's back. With his two hands he supports the two sides of the patient's lower jaw and slowly lifts. Then he bends the patient's head back to face upward. Where synovial inlay is suspected, it is most appropriate to use the neck-rotation method.

(ii) When the patient has an obvious traumatic history, and his injury involved great force, it is inadvisable to twist the neck suddenly when applying the neck-rotation method. Wait 2–3 days before using this part of the manipulation.

(iii) When no traumatic history is evident, but the symptoms are aggravated by exposure to wind and cold, it is advisable to perform more of the push and grasp massages, to grasp deeply and to knead heavily.

b) Other treatment: A typical case of torticollis will recover after two or three massage sessions. In general there is no need of other treatment. Where there is a traumatic history, a longer course of disability, or continued exposure to wind and cold, massage can be combined with the application of physical therapy, Chinese herbal lotions and local hot compresses.

Case History

Wu ——, male, age 34, worker. After he woke up one day he felt some soreness in the neck area. His symptoms became worse during the day until in late afternoon there was no free movement in the neck at all. He took an oral medication, but there was still no sign of improvement, so he came to the hospital for treatment. Examination: There was no redness or swelling in the neck, but tension of the neck muscles was noted. Pressure on the neck caused pain and pain arose from neck movement in any direction. After massage therapy, the pain was immediately diminished, and free movement returned. After the second treatment all symptoms completely vanished.

15. Acute Mastitis

Acute mastitis usually occurs post partum in breast-feeding women, especially with a first delivery. Doctors of Chinese medicine call it "out-blowing breast carbuncle." If the problem is not treated in time, it can form an abscess, which does not easily heal once it has burst.

Etiology

The origin of this disease is generally connected with a stagnant accumulation of lacteal fluid. Such an accumulation can take place either when regular feedings have not been possible or when the nipple is cracked and infection causes a blockage. The catabolins of the accumulated lacteal fluid stimulate the lactiferous ducts, giving rise to an inflammatory reaction. If the accumulation is not soon cleared, then the inflammation continues to develop, and a burst abscess is the end result.

Symptoms

A swelling pain is the only thing felt in the early stages. There is a swelling on the breast and a concealed swollen mass where mammary glands are blocked. The swollen mass gradually grows and becomes hard, and its boundary becomes more distinct. The skin in the area becomes red and the lymph nodes in the arm pit on the same side as the affected breast swell greatly. Finally the swollen mass becomes soft again, and turns into an abscess. Some burst spontaneously, exuding pus. After the onset, most patients have chills and fever.

Diagnosis

Based on the pathogenic process and local inflammation of the breast, it is easy to make a diagnosis. It is even easier when there is an abscess. However, if the mastitis progresses slowly, care must be taken to differentiate it from a breast tumor.

Treatment

Massage therapy should be applied at an early stage in the progress of this disease. Generally an abscess forms after 6–7 days, so it is advisable to apply massage before the abscess forms, as early as possible.

a) *Massage*: (i) The patient and the massage therapist sit facing each other. For a lubrication, smear the skin with a lubricating medium such as oil or talcum powder. First, the therapist lightly rubs and kneads around the lump in the breast. Some lacteal fluid will begin to drip out. Next, apply the dig and kneading methods to the *rugen* and *zhongfu* acupoints.

(ii) Then, supporting the breast with the fingers of both hands, use the two thumbs in alternation to rub down along the swollen mass from the top of the lump down to the nipple. Lacteal fluid will begin to spurt out. But the openings of the mammary glands on the side of the swollen mass will still be partly blocked, or all that comes out of them will be a small amount of yellow fluid.

(iii) With the left hand hold the breast firmly; with the thumb, index, and middle fingers of the right hand squeeze down along the swollen mass toward the nipple. Apply method (ii) alternately with this. The strength of the pinching is gradually increased to the extent that the patient can stand. From the openings of the occluded breast glands some creamy yellow liquid, or yellow pus-like liquid, will gradually be squeezed out. At this time the swollen mass will gradually become softer, or disperse. If no such effect takes place, then patiently keep on squeezing and rubbing. If the blockage has been partially opened up, but the patient cannot tolerate the pain, then rest for a while before beginning again. For the patient with severe pain, apply an analgesic prior to treatment.

b) *Other Treatment*: The breast can be held up with a broad belt and fomentations can be applied several times. At certain times, a breast pump or the hands can be used to empty out the lacteal fluid. Massage can be combined with the oral administration of Chinese herbal medicines for reducing inflammation and opening up the obstructed mammary ducts. If there is an excess of lacteal fluid, and the stagnant accumulation of it occurs again and again, then milk must be removed whenever necessary. Generally in Chinese folk-medicine, either Glauber's salt or leavened dough is wrapped in a piece of linen, and applied to the affected breast.

Therapeutic Effect

With massage treatment of acute mastitis, the earlier massage is begun the better. Generally, if the flow can be opened up in one session, the condition will clear up right away. If it cannot be opened up in one session, then a number of treatments will be necessary before the blockage slowly clears and the swollen mass dissipates completely. Where the condition has been present for a long time, and the flow cannot be opened up in one session, the therapeutic results of massage therapy are quite poor. Massage is generally not advisable where an abscess has formed and inflammation has spread over a relatively wide area.

Case History

Han ——, female, age 34, teacher. She was a woman who had given birth for the first time. Her right breast had been swollen and painful for two days and this had been accompanied by general fever for a day when she came for treatment. She said that feeding-times were irregular because she had to go to work, and that this caused the breast swelling to occur. For the past two days she had found a swollen mass and pain in her right breast. The previous day this had been accompanied by chills and fever. Examination: Body temperature 38 ° C. There was a red swollen mass on the upper part of her breast the size of a silver dollar. It was sore to the touch and the skin around it was slightly red. The condition was diagnosed as acute mastitis and massage therapy was given. After two massage sessions, the swollen mass disappeared, the skin color returned to normal and the lacteal fluid flowed unobstructedly. After a third session the symptoms completely disappeared and treatment was ended.

Note 1: Prescriptions for reducing inflammation and opening the mammary ducts:

a) *Pugongying*	Taraxacum mongolicum Hand.-Mazz. (dandelion)	1 *liang*
Jinyinhua	Lonicera japonica Thunb. (honeysuckle flower)	1 *liang*
Gualou (whole)	Trichosanthes kirilowii Maxim.	5 *qian*
Mutong	Akebia trifoliata (Thunb.) Koidz. (fruit)	5 *qian*

The above herbs are decocted in three Chinese bowls of water until only one bowl of liquid remains. This is taken orally.

b) *Pugongying*	Taraxacum mongolicum Hand.-Mazz. (dandelion)	1 *liang*
Zihuadiding	Viola japonica Langsd.	1 *liang*

Decocted in water and taken orally.

Note 2: *Folk Massage Method—Scraping with a wooden comb:* Use a wooden comb, preferably an old, smooth one. Dip the back of the comb into sesame oil and use it to scrape over the swollen mass of the breast down in the direction of the nipple, gradually increasing the amount of force used. At this time the lacteal fluid will flow out. Repeat patiently until milk flows smoothly from the occluded mammary ducts.

Note 3: *Folk Massage—The tread-pull method:* Have the patient take a sitting position, with the practitioner sitting on the patient's affected side. With the foot against the patient's armpit, grasp the patient's fingers with both hands. Simultaneously push against the armpit and pull on the hand. Repeat 3–4 times. Grasp different combinations of fingers each time. For instance, during the first tread-pull movement the right hand may hold the thumb and index fingers, while the left hand holds the other three fingers; then during the second tread-pull movement, the right hand holds the thumb, index, and middle fingers and the left hand holds the other two fingers. After a series of tread-pull movements, the patient should feel a relaxing, comfortable sensation in the breast area.

16. Thromboangiitis Obliterans

Etiology

The causes of this disease have not yet been confirmed, but it is generally thought that it may be connected with factors such as smoking, drinking, cold, and psychological factors. Owing to the above factors an imbalance is created in the central nervous system that results in spasm of the arteries. Long-term angiospasm results in such pathologic changes as thickening of the inner lining of the blood vessels, blood-clot formation, and even complete blockage. At the same time a set of corresponding symptoms appears clinically.

Symptoms

This disease usually occurs in one of the lower limbs. In the early stages chills and numbness are felt in the affected limb and there is often an indefinite aching in the calf and the foot. When the condition is somewhat more serious, what is called "intermittent claudication" appears; walking only a short distance causes pain and muscle spasms in the calf which together force the patient to limp. After a short rest, the pain vanishes, but walking for a short while causes the symptoms to arise again. As the condition reaches its later stages, the patient feels an obvious coolness of the affected limb, and the toes are in constant pain. This often causes the patient to sit hugging his knees, in order to relieve the pain somewhat. The pain is often worse at night and when the leg is raised. The skin grows purplish-red and the patient cannot work at all. Should the condition continue to develop, ulcers and necrosis appear in the leg, especially in the toes.

Diagnosis

This is not difficult to diagnose, based on the specific symptoms and further inquiry about other factors such as smoking, drinking, exposure to cold, and psychological factors. Early discovery and treatment is most important.

Treatment

a) Massage: (i) The patient lies face down. First apply the flat-thumb push to the low back and sacral areas and massage the *shenshu*, *mingmen*, and the eight *liao* acupoints, chiefly using the thumb-tip push method. Then apply the roll method, starting at the gluteal area and going down toward the affected leg. Alternate this with going upward from the calf using the flat-palm push. Alternate the two methods 3–4 times. Do not massage too long and do not massage hard enough to cause pain.

(ii) The patient lies on his back. Apply the flat-palm push method going up along the calf and thigh. Then go downward using the roll method. Alternate the two methods 3–4 times.

(iii) Then exert pressure with the thumbs on either side of the *qichong* acupoint. After about 2–3 minutes, the patient will say he feels a numb, swelling sensation in the leg. At this point, suddenly release the thumbs. The patient will feel a stream of warmth rush downward. Doing this once or twice is enough. If it causes severe pain, do not do it at all.

(iv) Finally, gently vibrate the affected limb 1–2 minutes with the palm or with a vibrator.

a) Other Treatment: Massage is only part of an effective combined treatment for this disease. Both clinical administration of medication and surgical treatment are also important. Other measures such as abstaining from smoking and drinking, keeping the affected limb warm, and doing appropriate medical exercise must also not be neglected.

Case History

Li ——, male, age 32, elementary school teacher. In the lower end of the left calf, and in the toe area of the left foot an aching pain had set in three years before while he was walking. Intermittent claudication was present following the gradual development of his condition. Recently, a spasmodic pain had developed in the affected limb, becoming more severe at night. At the same time he had a cold numb feeling. Examination: The skin in the calf and foot of the affected leg was dark and red, and colder than the right leg. The pulse in the artery in the instep of the left foot was weak. The pain remained unchanged when the leg was raised or allowed to hang down. Thromboangiitis obliterans was diagnosed. After the use of the above-mentioned methods of massage and medical exercise, at each session the pain diminished, and the skin became flushed. Thereafter, with clinical applications of lumbar and femoral sympathetic ganglion nerve block therapy added, treatment continued for a total of 44 days. By then, all the symptoms were completely gone and the patient was discharged.

17. Postoperative Paralytic Intestinal Obstruction

Etiology

This condition occurs most often after abdominal surgery. It is related to the violent stimulation of the surgery, including that of the anesthetic. General functional disturbance is caused by this stimulation, and a temporary disturbance of peristaltic function appears.

Symptoms

It usually sets in 1–3 days after the operation. Abdominal distention is gradually felt. There is no passing of flatus and no desire for a bowel movement. The distention of the abdomen gradually becomes so bad that breathing may be affected and lying flat is not possible. The patient shows annoyance and impatience, and serious cases cannot sleep. He or she has no appetite or desire to drink, and vomiting appears. During examination the distention of the abdomen can be seen and percussion of the abdomen produces a sound like a drum. The peristaltic sound is found to be very weak, or nonexistent.

Diagnosis

It is not difficult to diagnose this condition by etiology and symptoms. But massage therapy can be applied only after all the general contraindications are eliminated.

Treatment

a) Massage: (i) Have the patient turn slowly onto his/her side. The flat-thumb push method is applied to both sides of the middle section of the back area (from the lower section of the chest to the upper section of the lumbar region) for about 5 minutes, in order to make the patient feel familiar with the massage stimulation, and comfortable.

(ii) With the thumb apply the dig method to both of the *pishu* and *weishu* acupoints till the vital energy appears. Then the thumb kneading method is applied to each acupoint for about 1 minute, so as to maintain the strength of the stimulation. At this time the patient often feels a peristalsis in his abdomen, or an immediate flatus. With no such reaction, the finger dig and thumb-kneading methods can be applied above and below the *pishu* and *weishu* points, or a sensitive point on the back can be used as an *ashi*[1] point.

(iii) The patient lies on his/her back. Apply the palm-rub method to the navel, moving clockwise. At this time there is often a peristaltic sensation, the patient may produce flatus, and the distention of the abdomen may gradually subside. Should the effect not become apparent, then apply the finger-dig and finger-vibrate methods to the *tianshu* and *qihai* acupoints, following the rise and fall of respiration. Finally conclude by kneading and rubbing the abdomen firmly with the flat of the palm.

b) Other treatment: Aside from the above methods of massage, other symptomatic treatments should be applied at the same time, such as decompression by gastro-intubation and insertion of a tube into the anus for passing flatus, to promote the recovery of peristaltic function.

Therapeutic Effect

Generally, massage has a quick effect upon this condition. Sometimes all the symptoms almost completely vanish after one session of massage.

Case History

Du ——, male, age 40, cadre. Outside consultation. The patient suffered from chronic appendicitis. The third day after surgical treatment his ab-

---

1. *ashi* points—Any point on the body that is not an acupoint, but to which acupoint massage is applied. It is often done near the site of an injury.

domen was highly distended. He could not eat or drink, passed no flatus, gave no sign of bowel movement, and auscultation of the abdomen showed that the peristaltic sound had disappeared. It was clinically diagnosed to be postoperative intestinal paralysis. By gastro-intubation, insertion of a tube into the anus, and injection of neostigmine, no recovery of peristalsis was obtained. The above methods of massage were adopted. After the *pishu* acupoint on the right side was massaged by the finger dig and thumb kneading methods for one minute, the patient felt peristaltic movement. After massaging the left *pishu* acupoint in the same way, the passing of flatus took place. At the end of the massage the patient expelled a large amount of gas, and suddenly felt relaxed and comfortable in his abdominal region. The next day he was re-examined. The distention in the abdomen had disappeared. No further treatment was given.

18. Paraplegia

Paraplegia is a general term for paralytic symptoms in the lower half of the body. Massage therapy is one of the comparatively positive methods in the comprehensive treatment of paraplegia.

Etiology

Paraplegia can occur in a great number of conditions, such as spinal fracture, spondylo-tuberculosis concurrent with myelolesion, myelitis, myeloma, etc.

Symptoms

Paraplegia can occur suddenly or gradually. The location of the paralysis, high or low, is normally determined by the location of the pathological changes. There can be motor disturbances and sensory disturbances at the site of the paralysis. The motor disturbances may involve partial or complete loss of motor ability; the sensory disturbances may include sensory retardation, sensory anomaly, superficial and deep sensory losses. Based on the different degrees of motor and sensory disturbance, a clinical distinction is made between complete and incomplete paralysis. In addition, paraplegia can also display either spastic paralysis or flaccid paralysis. In spastic paralysis the muscles at the paralysed site are spasmodic, the muscle-tension increases, atrophy is not apparent, and there are pathological reflexes. In flaccid paralysis the muscles at the site of paralysis become loose, soft, and asthenic, their tension decreases, there is obvious muscular atrophy, and all the various reflexes weaken or disappear.

Diagnosis

It is not hard to diagnose paraplegia, but the causes of the condition are comparatively complex, and must be clearly identified. It is only paraplegia resulting from lesion or inflammation that can be successfully treated by clinical management including massage therapy. In paraplegia arising from other causes, this treatment has a relatively poor therapeutic effect. In treatment of paraplegia caused by tumor, massage must only be adopted after treating the tumor. Prior to the employment of massage therapy, a distinction between spastic paralysis and flaccid paralysis must be made, because the types of massage therapy used are somewhat different.

Treatment

The therapist and the patient must first establish firm confidence that they can overcome the paraplegia. Then they actively select massage methods to combine with other forms of clinical treatment. The choice of methods is based on the stage of development of the paraplegia and on its clinical manifestations.

a) *Massage*: (i) The patient first takes a natural lying position. His limbs rest in suitable positions. Sometimes the limbs have to be exposed and a lubricating medium applied.

(ii) At the beginning of a massage session, take special care to make your movements steady and even, increasing pressure from light to heavy. Generally, the first methods used are the circular rub, push and rub. Gradually switch from these to the kneading method, kneading from distal to proximal, and for about 5–10 minutes.

(iii) In cases of spastic paralysis, be particularly sure that your movements are steady and even, and that the massage does not go too deep. Gradually use more force, according to the patient's gradual adaptation to the stimulation. The amount of force used should normally not be so great as to cause spastic contractions.

(iv) In cases of flaccid paralysis, the massage can be heavier, reaching right down into the muscles. The pinch method can be employed, using three fingers or five, depending on the area to be massaged. Pinch and knead the muscles at the site of paralysis deeply. On some areas, strong manipulations such as the flick method can be applied, and the rub-roll method can be utilized as well. Finally, various forms of the hammer and pat methods can be used.

(v) Adopt acupoint massage. Based on the high or low position of the paralysed site, select acupoints such as *qichong, huantiao, juliao, fengshi, zusanli, yanglingquan, xuehai, weizhong, chengshan, taixi, kunlun* and *jiexi*. To all of these, the finger-dig and finger-vibrate methods can be applied, and especially the thumb-tip push method, which is applied most to the *zusanli* point.

(vi) It is very important to apply passive massage manipulations to the patient with complete paralysis. Before active movement is restored, passive manipulations such as flexing and extending the joints can be used to promote the building up in the motor organs of the various conditions for movement. Generally, this should be done several times every day. At the same time, positive use should be made of methods that stimulate movement, in order to promote the occurrence and restoration of active movement. Have the patient lie on his side. The therapist supports the patient's leg with one arm, bending each joint of the leg as much as possible. The therapist tells the patient to extend the leg and gently moves each joint to the extended position, following the force exerted by the patient. Repeated use of such methods of stimulating movement can help the patient to recover active movement.

(vii) For the patient who is incontinent of feces or urine, kneading or rubbing massage can be applied to the abdomen. At the same time apply acupoint massage to the *guanyuan, qihai*, and *tianshu* points on the abdomen or the *dachangshu, xiaochangshu* and eight *liao* points on the back. Acupoint massage will gradually promote restoration of eliminative function.

b) *Other treatment*: During the entire course of treatment, massage should be combined with various effective new treatments involving drugs, acupuncture, and injections of herbal medicines. When active movement begins to reappear, a program of medical exercise should be instituted. While the muscles are still not strong enough to overcome the weight of the limb itself, it is best to use a weight and pulley to reduce the weight of the limb while various forms of exercise are carried out. In setting up an exercise program, special attention has to be paid to developing a positive attitude on the part of the patient. Under the guidance of the therapist, he or she will be undertaking an arduous training program. At the same time the patient should frequently perform active relaxation exercises for the limbs.

In the medical exercise the body position the patient takes has to be moved as fast as possible toward the transition to standing up and walking. When the patient is in a lying position, frequently stimulate his plantar area, and apply passive manipulations that stimulate walking. He can also practice standing with the help of mechanical aids. For example, use a plank bed with one end fixed on the ground and the other placed higher. The patient lies on it with his feet against a fixed transverse board. The elevation of the higher end of the plank bed is gradually increased until the patient is just about standing straight. When he can stand up he can learn to walk supported by another person, by a cane or with a high stool. Where conditions permit, a walking cart can also be used.

Therapeutic Effect

In the early stages of paralysis massage therapy can raise the body's resistance, prevent bed sores, and stop retrogressive changes such as atrophy of a motor organ or articular ankylosis, and has the function of promoting the reappearance and development of active movement. When the paralysed patient has recovered some active movement, massage therapy can help him to stand and develop his ability to walk sooner.

Case History No. 1

Liu ——, male, age 50, cadre. The patient first felt numbness and weakness in the lower limbs. After two or three days both legs were so completely paralysed that he could not walk. After having lain in bed for about a week he came to the neurology department of our hospital, and was hospitalized for treatment. His condition was diagnosed to be a traverse myelitis. He was immediately given massage therapy. At that time his lower limbs could not be actively moved, any sensation of pain had completely disappeared from the thigh down and the muscles were weak and slightly atrophied. The knee reflex was gone and there was no pathological reflex. Therefore the massage therapy for flaccid paralysis was adopted. After one week of treatment active movement in the lower limbs was basically restored. He could bend his knees and make a slight straight-leg elevation. The treatment was continued for a week, and after the addition of active medical exercise, movement in the lower limbs was completely recovered, and he could get out of bed and stand up. Measurement of the circumference of his legs revealed no diminution, but rather an increase since the beginning of massage. He was discharged from hospital and convalesced at home.

Case History No. 2

Fang ——, male, age 25, soldier. The patient had tuberculosis of the 8th to 10th thoracic vertebrae, with paraplegia, and was hospitalized for treatment. Examination: His lower limbs were found to be hyperesthetic. There was no obvious atrophy in the muscles. The muscles in the thigh could be actively contracted a slight amount. There was no movement at all from the calves to the toes, but in the whole lower limb there was an involuntary tremor, as well as pathological reflex. Therefore a cleanup operation on the tuberculous focus was performed in the Division of Orthopedics. Five days after the first operation, the massage therapy for spastic paralysis was begun. This was intended to help restore some movement in the paralysed lower limbs, and to make the knees able to bend and extend fully. After a month and a half of massage treatment, a second operation was performed. After the surgery, massage treatment was continued. At the same time the patient was given a program of medical exercise for the lower limbs. After a stay in hospital of over 4 months in all, and over 100 massage sessions, function was basically restored in the lower limbs. When he could walk almost normally, the patient was discharged.

19. Partial Paralysis

Partial paralysis is also called hemiplegia. The word is a general term for paralytic symptoms that occur on one side of the body. This condition is most common in old age. Massage therapy has a positive therapeutic effect.

Etiology

Clinically, hemiplegia can occur concurrently with a great number of diseases, e.g. head injury, cerebral angiopathy, intracranial tumor, etc. Clinically, the hemiplegia resulting from hypertensive cerebral hemorrhage (stroke) is the most common.

Symptoms

Hemiplegia usually comes on suddenly, though a minority of cases are gradual. There are motor and sensory disturbances of one side of the patient's body, and often slanting of the mouth and eye. Hemiplegia is generally a form of spastic paralysis, but in its early stages there may be a period during which it manifests itself as flaccid paralysis. The degree of motor and sensory disturbance shown can represent either complete paralysis or incomplete paralysis.

Diagnosis

A positive diagnosis can generally be made on the basis of symptoms, but the etiology of the hemiplegia, including the disease that gave rise to it, must be determined.

Treatment

Massage therapy is normally begun after the hemiplegia has been dealt with clinically, when the pathogenic factors have been eliminated or the patient's condition stabilized, and the patient's mind has become clearer. In the course of treatment great attention must be paid to overcoming the patient's passive mood and strengthening his confidence for the battle with his condition.

a) *Massage*: (i) The patient lies flat. Circular rub, push and rub manipulations are applied to the limbs on the paralyzed side going from light to heavy, and from the extremity towards the trunk of the limb. Massage evenly for 5–10 minutes. If there is still some high blood pressure this treatment can be combined with systemic massage and other methods used for treatment of hypertension. (See page 187.)

(ii) Hemiplegia is generally spastic paralysis, but in its early stages it manifests itself as flaccid paralysis, and should be treated as such. Use the massage methods for flaccid paralysis described in the section on treatment of paraplegia. (See page 167.)

(iii) Acupoint massage. For acupoints on the lower limbs, see the section on treatment of paraplegia (page 167). On the upper limbs, the *quepen, jianliao, jianjing, quchi, chize, shaohai, daling, yangchi, yangxi, yanggu, shousanli,* and *hegu* acupoints are commonly used, with the finger dig and finger vibrate massage methods. Emphasis can be placed on applying the thumb-tip push to the *shousanli* and *hegu* acupoints.

(iv) Before there is active movement, the patient's healthy limbs can be used for assisted exercise. The healthy hand can pull the affected hand; the healthy foot can support the affected foot. The therapist and the patient's family can help him to exercise the affected limb. Much use can be made of the movement-stimulation method: The therapist or a member of the patient's family supports the affected limb. The therapist tells the patient to move the affected limb, at the same time moving it for him. The patient himself consciously exerts force on the limb, gradually establishing active movement. A movement-stimulation method for the lower limbs is described in the section on treatment of paraplegia. (See page 167.)

(v) If there is slanting of the mouth and eye, rubbing and kneeding massage of the paralysed side of the face can be used. The thumb-tip push can also be applied to the *taiyang, zuanzhu, jingming, yifeng, jiache,* and *dicang* acupoints.

b) *Other Treatment:* Methods of treatment such as drugs, acupuncture and moxibustion, etc., must be applied in conjunction. After the patient has some active movement, medical exercise should be started as soon as possible. Generally, the active movement in the lower limb will be restored before that in the upper limb. Therefore the change should be made as soon as possible to more active postures. A movement-stimulation method for the upper limbs can be performed with the patient either sitting or standing. The upper limb on the affected side can be moved toward the shoulder on the healthy side. The head and neck can also be turned as far as possible toward the healthy side. At the therapist's oral command, the head, neck, and trunk are turned toward the affected side. At the same time, the therapist carries the affected arm toward the affected side and consciously extends the whole upper limb, exerting force right to the fingers. This process is repeated a number of times. When the upper limb regains mobility, coordinated movement should be exercised as early as possible. For example, have the two hands alternately point at the nose and touch the ears, and have the two upper limbs alternately make movements in different directions. At the same time have the patient practice practical movements such as eating with chopsticks and writing with a pen. In addition, active relaxation exercise for the muscles of the affected limb should be done frequently.

Therapeutic Effect

Massage therapy has a positive effect on promoting the restoration of mobility in the hemiplegic patient. If in the later stages of the disease it is combined with medical exercise, therapeutic effect is even better.

Case History

Fang ———, male, age 55, worker. The patient suddenly collapsed and his mind became confused. Later, partial paralysis appeared on his left side. After a month, he had recovered clarity of mind and was basically able to talk again. But he could not move the limbs on the left side of his body at all. In addition to medication, massage was applied as above. The total number of massage treatments was 30. Movement was gradually restored to the limbs on his left side. The muscles were strong enough to move the limbs, and he could walk with something to support him. He was told to continue with massage and medical exercise after he was discharged from hospital.

20. Peripheral Nerve Bundle Injury

After a peripheral nerve bundle injury various degrees of paralysis can be present in limbs below the injury. Massage therapy can have definite results, as part of a combined treatment.

Etiology

Peripheral nerve bundle injury is usually seen at the time of injury to the soft tissues (by cutting, puncture, contusion by a blunt instrument, etc.) or of fracture. It can also be caused by accidental injury to the nerve trunk during surgery or by surgical excision of neurofibroma, etc.

Symptoms

After the injury, motor and sensory disturbances usually appear immediately in areas corresponding to those controlled by the damaged nerves. Mild disturbance involves only numbness, decrease in muscle tone and weakened mobility. In severe disturbance, both sensation and active muscle contraction are lost and there is deformation and spasm in the affected limb. The paralysis brought on by perineural injury is always flaccid paralysis. The site of the paralysis is clearly delimited by the site of the injured nerve trunk. Therefore we have clinical designations such as neural injury to the brachial plexus, the radial nerve, the ulnar nerve, the femoral nerve, or the common peroneal nerve.

Diagnosis

This condition is comparatively easy to diagnose on the basis of symptoms and traumatic history. But the area that is actually injured must be clearly distinguished, so that the appropriate massage therapy can be adopted. Distinctions in muscle-strength are also relevant: in clinical practice it is important to know whether there is active muscle-contraction and the strength of muscle resistance.

Treatment

Surgical management is necessary in some cases but not in others. In those that do not require surgery, massage therapy can be applied as early as possible.

a) Massage (i) Body position: Use a sitting position for an injury to an upper limb, and a lying position for one to a lower limb. Put the limb to be massaged in an appropriate position. Expose as much as possible the site that needs massaging, and apply a lubricating medium.

(ii) First apply the knead and rub methods to the limb. Then gradually increase the amount of force used, carrying the massage deeper and deeper. Then the three-finger and five-finger pinch methods are applied focusing on the paralysed muscle group. The roll method can be applied to the thigh and other parts of the body whose area is comparatively large. At the same time the roll and pinch methods are being applied, various kinds of passive manipulations can be performed on the joints of the paralysed limb, especially movements in the opposite direction to the contractions of the antagonistic muscles.

(iii) Based on different sites of paralysis select corresponding acupoints: e.g. for an ulnar nerve paralysis select *quchi*, *chize*, *shousanli*, *waiguan*, and *hegu*, and apply the finger dig, finger vibrate and thumb-tip push methods. A strong stimulation has to be applied, but only for a short time.

(iv) In serious cases with no active muscle contraction, movement-stimulation methods can be part of the treatment. For instance, when the extensor muscles of the forearm are paralysed, the therapist bends the patient's elbow, wrist, and fingers as far as possible, then tells him/her to consciously try to extend the whole arm, while the therapist moves the forearm and fingers to the extended position. This helps stimulate the reappearance of active movement.

(v) Finally, the massage session is concluded by kneading and rubbing the paralysed limb once or twice. The whole course of massage should not be overly long, around 15 minutes. However, it is best to repeat it 2–3 times a day. Teach the patient's family how to carry out the above method of massage with him.

b) *Other Treatment:* At the same time such treatments as acupuncture, Chinese herbal medicines, physical therapy, etc., can be adopted in order to heighten therapeutic effect. Medical exercise can be used in cases where the muscles already have active movement. The principle of the medical exercise method should be to forcefully exercise the muscles of the affected limb in every direction, alternating with the sound limb. The patient has to be encouraged to exert as much force as possible. Each exercise session should not be too long, and proper rest should be taken. In cases where the patient's muscles are not strong enough, an exercise method that reduces the weight of the limbs may be used. One simple method is to have the patient lie on his or her side, with the limb on a smooth, flat surface. This makes active movement, such as bending and extending, easy.

A weight and pulley can also be employed to reduce the weight of the affected limb, or the limb can be gently supported by the practitioner, so that its weight is reduced. Later on, as the muscles become stronger, gradually lessen the weight on the pulley or the amount of support given by the practitioner.

Therapeutic Effect

The application of massage therapy following peripheral neural injury can improve blood circulation, prevent muscular atrophy, and stimulate reappearance and development of active movement. Certain cases require surgery, and in these postoperative massage therapy can often obtain a satisfactory result.

Case History

Wang——, male, age 30, cadre. The patient was hospitalized for treatment of neurofibroma in his right armpit, and a neurectomy and nerve anastomosis were performed. His knee joint was fixed at 90 degrees after the operation Two weeks after surgery the immobility began to be relieved, but the knee still could not extend straight. A flaccid paralysis was present in the leg. Use was made of massage in combination with the appropriate amount of passive traction and medical exercise. After 40-days' treatment the flaccid paralysis was obviously improved. The knee could be extended straight and the patient was able to walk with a cane. He was instructed to continue massage and medical exercise after he was discharged.

21. Infantile Paralysis

Infantile paralysis is also called poliomyelitis. The specific signs include general symptoms and acute flare-ups of flaccid paralysis.

Etiology

This is an infantile infectious disease due to a particular species of filtrable virus infection. It is common in one- to six-year-old children. The patient's feces and nasopharyngeal secretions contain large amounts of the virus, chiefly passed by dietary infection. Aside from this, saliva passing through the mouth and a wound in the skin can also lead to infection. This disease is mostly seen at the end of summer and the beginning of autumn.

Symptoms

Aside from a latent period, the course of this disease may generally be divided into three phases.:

(i) Premonitory phase: Fever of 38–40°C, general discomfort, headache, and pharyngeal pain, accompanied by symptoms in the digestive system, such as anorexia, abdominal pain, diarrhea, and vomiting. Fever diminishes after 1–4 days and the symptoms completely disappear. At this period there are no symptoms in the nervous system.

(ii) Pre-paralytic phase: 1–6 days after the fever of the premonitory period disappears, fever recurs. The whole body shows excitation and pain is experienced all over the body or in the limbs. The patient rejects any type of caress offered by others. Sensation is hypersensitive. The muscles at the back of the neck are spasmodic and tetanic. The various tendon reflexes remain normal or increase. The patient's mind is usually clear.

(iii) Paralytic phase: The above-mentioned symptoms persist for 3–10 days. Then the fever begins to rise. During the period of the fever, or after it subsides, a flaccid paralysis appears and gradually becomes accentuated.. Often the reflex of the abdominal wall is the first to disappear, and the knee reflex gradually weakens to the point of disappearance. Generally, the fever drops after 5–10 days and the paralysis goes no further. The paralysis is usually found in the limbs, particularly in the lower limbs. Paralysis of the head and trunk is less common.

Diagnosis

(i) Premonitory phase: Lay stress on noticing the endemic conditions in a community. It is very hard to make a definite diagnosis.

(ii) Pre-paralytic phase: If there is stiffness in the neck a lumbar puncture should be performed at once, examining the cerebro-spinal fluid in order to be sure the problem is not meningitis.

(iii) Paralytic phase: The following points should be noted: The paralysis is flaccid paralysis; its distribution is uneven and completely asymmetrical;

sometimes it appears in one muscle or one group of muscles. There is a history of fever before the paralysis sets in. At an early stage of paralysis, there are clear changes in the cerebro-spinal fluid; sometimes, although the white blood cell count is down, there is a clear increase in globulin.

Treatment

a) *Massage*: Paralysis of the lower limbs is used as an example: (i) Have the patient lie on his/her back. When massaging use as a medium the medicinal wine for infantile paralysis. (See p. 78.) The practitioner begins by supporting the child's heel with his right hand; with his left thumb and middle finger he pinches and twists from the sides of the toe to the end of the toe. Then with his thumb he pushes along the tendons of the top of the foot. He repeats this for each toe in the same order. The process is repeated 10 times or more, for about two minutes.

(ii) With the flat of the thumb encircle the lateral condyle of the ankle joint and apply a circular rubbing to it for about 1 minute. Do the same to the medial condyle also for about 1 minute.

(iii) With the left hand supporting the heel of the child's foot and the right hand tightly against the ends of the toes, apply passive manipulation to the ankle joint, bending and extending it. Apply force to bend it and relax to extend.

(iv) With the knee of the affected limb bent, knead the *xiyan* acupoint for 1-2 minutes, using both thumbs. Then rub around the knee joint with the flats of both palms.

(v) With the thumb apply a push massage to the muscle group in front of the tibia about 30-50 times.

(vi) Alternating right and left hands, apply a push massage to the medial and lateral muscle groups of the thigh and to the anterior thigh muscles. If there is any abduction or outward rotation of the calf, apply a heavy pinch massage to the muscle groups of the medial thigh, for about 3 minutes.

(vii) With the left hand supporting the child's calf, use the right palm to apply a push massage to the whole leg. When pushing use heavy force; when coming back use light force. Do this about 80-100 times.

(viii) With the patient lying face down, use the thumbs to apply the finger kneading method along both sides of the spinal column with some force, going up the spinal column about 10 times. Then use the two thumbs to massage outward from both sides of the spinal column in the divergent push method, several tens of times.

(ix) The spinal pinch method is applied upward along the two sides of the vetebral column. Pinch until a slight redness appears. (See Diagram 79.) Then do a heavy dig at both *huantiao* acupoints and in the area of the greater trochanter for 2–3 minutes. The strength of the stimulation must be great.

(x) Use the two-palm pat method, lightly patting for about 1 minute from the vetebral column down toward the heel. Then use the palms to push along the back and the thigh.

(xi) With three fingers pinch the back of the leg, going up and down several tens of times.

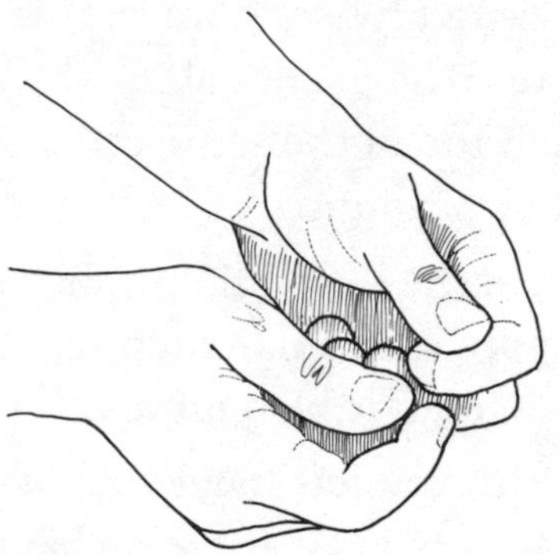

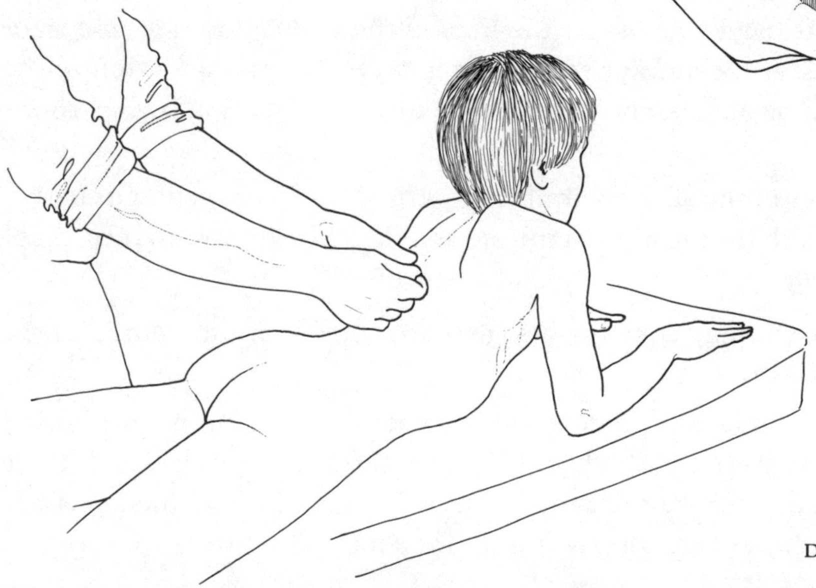

DIAGRAM 79

(xii) Using thumb and index finger, apply the grasp method to the Achilles tendon for about 1–2 minutes. Again with the thumb apply the dig massage to acupoints such as *chengshan*, *weizhong*, *zusanli*, and *yinlingquan*.

(xiii) Finally, gently push up and down the back of the thigh.

b) *Other treatment:* Other treatments such as acupuncture, physical therapy, and medical exercise can be used in combination with massage therapy.

Therapeutic Effect

In infantile paralysis, massage prevents muscular atrophy, promotes restoration of mobility, and has the possible effect of correcting deformation. Therapeutic effect is high on cases in their early stages, but comparatively low on those in their later stages. In advanced cases where the deformative aftereffects of infantile paralysis are already evident, massage therapy is ineffective. Massage can also be used before and after surgery to correct deformities.

Case History

Zhang ——, female, 15 months old. The affected child suddenly had a high fever. After three days the fever ceased. But it was discovered that she could not stand on her right leg. She was afraid to have any adult rub it. After half a month, because she could not move her right leg at all, she came to the hospital for treatment. Infantile paralysis was diagnosed after examination in the Pediatric Division. Massage therapy was applied. At this time there was no active movement at all in the lower limb on the affected side. The muscles in the calf and thigh were completely flaccid and without strength. After one week of treatment, there was some movement in the thigh muscles and an automatic bend-extend movement in the ankle, and she could stand independently for a little while. After half a month of treatment she could already begin to move about. At this time the quadriceps and adductor muscles of the thigh, as well as the muscle group in the calf in front of the tibia, were all asthenic. Therefore, a deep pinch was applied to the muscles in those areas. After 40 massage treatments, there was some progress in the strength of the muscles of the calf and thigh. Outward rotation of the leg and plantar flexion were greatly improved, to the point that she could walk by herself for about ten paces. Treatment was stopped, but her family was instructed to continue giving her massage and walking-practice.

22. Contracture

Contracture is a symptom rather than a disease. The sustained contraction of a muscle group of the body resulting from any cause is called "contracture." There is contracture due to inflammation, diminution in blood supply, paralysis, scar etc.; flexive contracture of the hip and knee joints caused by an abscess in the iliac fossa; or suppurative osteoarthritis of the hip; contracture due to lack of blood supply in the upper limbs or subsequent to arterial blood transfusion; contracture of the antagonistic muscle during infantile paralysis; and scar contracture after burn.

Symptoms and Diagnosis

Contracture is most likely to occur in the limbs. The muscles of the contracted part will be extremely tense. When the limb is pulled straight, there will be some sense of resistance, and perhaps pain, so that the mobility of the contracted joint is impeded. But the joint will not be ankylotic. In diagnosing contracture, its cause must also be identified.

Treatment

Massage is used only as a symptomatic treatment. The cause of the contracture must be found and dealt with at the same time.

a) *Massage:* (i) The palm-heel rub method or the thumb rub method is first applied to the contracted part. Then the knead and pinch methods are used, going from shallow to deep and massaging for 3–5 minutes.

(ii) Acupoint massage for the upper limbs, using as massage points *jianyu*, *quchi*, *shaohai*, *hegu*, and *neiguan*. For the lower limbs use the *xuehai*, *weizhong*, *chengshan*, *chengjin* (situated above *chengshan*, in the middle of the gastrocnemius muscle) and *taixi* acupoints. Start with acupoints at the joint nearest the contracture, then move to those further away. Apply the dig and kneading methods for about 1 minute each time, until the vital energy is tapped.

(iii) Traction. The force applied in pulling straight the contracted muscles must be firm and steady. It should be gradually increased, but violence must be avoided. At the same time as the muscles are pulled straight, massage is applied to the contracted muscle group and to acupoints at the nearest joint. Knead and pinch the contracted muscle group or dig the points in the vicinity of the joint, and pull it out straight at the same time. The scope of the extension is increased daily, but without rushing. When the limb has been extended to a certain point, keep it there for 1–2 minutes.

(iv) Finally, apply knead, pinch, rub-roll, and vibrate massages to the muscle groups of the contracted part for 1–2 minutes.

b) *Other Treatments:* Other treatments should be applied in accordance with the cause of contracture. Acupuncture and physiotherapy can help to eliminate the contractive symptoms.

Therapeutic Effect

The effectiveness of massage in treatment of contracture depends largely on the cause of the contracture and the length of time for which contracture has been present. Generally speaking, therapeutic effect is more satisfactory when treatment is applied early.

Case History No. 1

Zhang ——, male, age 23, farmer. Because of a swollen mass and pain in the inguinalis region of the right thigh, the mobility of the right hip joint was restricted, with the accompaniment of fever all over the body. The patient was examined in the Surgery Department. He was diagnosed to have an abscess of the right iliac fossa. He was hospitalized and underwent surgery, during which the abscess was opened and drained. The infection was under control after about a month and a half. The local incision drained freely, but flexive contracture of the right hip and knee joints appeared, with greatest extension 160 degrees. Massage therapy was given, combined with medical exercise. In the late stages of treatment skin traction was applied. After 8 treatment sessions, the hip and knee joints's extension was very close to normal.

Case History No. 2

Du ——, female, age 19, farmer. The top third of the left humerus and the top third of the left femur were openly fractured. She was sent to the hospital for emergency treatment, in the course of which a blood transfusion into the right radial artery was given. Her right hand and the muscle group of her forearm showed obvious contracture. Active movement functions in the wrist and other joints were obviously impeded. After seven massage-therapy sessions, the contracture was clearly improved, and mobility in the joints approached normal.

23. Decubitus Ulcer (Bedsore)

Decubitus ulcer is a type of necrotic ulcer in the soft tissue. It is often seen in a bed-ridden patient with a weak constitution. Once bedsore is formed the ulcerated part heals extremely slowly. Serious decubitus ulcers can even bring about septicemia causing death.

Etiology

The patient who is bed-ridden for long periods of time, especially one who is unable to change position, will develop bedsores due to local malnutrition when the weight of the body puts pressure on an area of skin, subcutaneous tissue, and other soft tissues, leading to poor blood circulation and impeded supply of nutrients.

Symptoms

In the early stages, there are usually no subjective symptoms. By the time the patient feels discomfort and sharp local pain, the ulcer has usually already formed.

Diagnosis

The patient's constitution is usually quite weak. The bedsores occur at the points on which the body is supported, such as the shoulder blade, sacrum, heel, and elbow. At the early stages the skin appears dark and red, without lustre, and lacks elasticity. There is a slight pain when the skin in pressed. In the later stages, the skin undergoes tissue death, and an ulcer is formed. The surface of the ulcer is filthy with a mixture of exudates, and may even be open to the bone. Sometimes the ulcer may infiltrate the surrounding subcutaneous tissues, forming a pocket-like ulcer.

Treatment

a) Massage: In massage treatment of decubitus ulcer, different conditions call for the adoption of different methods of massage, which are separately described below:

(i) Preventive measures: The patient who is bed-ridden for a long period of time, especially the paralytic patient must start to receive prophylactic massage as early as possible. The massage is concentrated on the areas of the body that are under pressure, but general massage of the whole body is given as well. Normally, the palm-base circular-rub method is adopted, following the direction of the blood flow. The manipulation is increased from light to heavy. The effect of the massage will be improved by dipping the palm into medicinal liquor before massaging.

(ii) Massage for bedsores in their early stages: Generally, the thumb or the fleshy pad at the base of the thumb can be employed to apply the circular rub method, rubbing from the center of the bedsore toward its circumference, so that the blood that has collected in the area is dispersed. This in turn promotes re-supply with fresh, new blood, turning the skin from dark to red. At this point, although an ulcer has not yet formed, skin is poorly supplied with nutrients, and easily broken, so massage must be light and dexterous. General massage and passive manipulations of the limbs must also be intensified.

(iii) Massage for bedsores in their later stages: Since an ulcer has already formed at this point, the effect of the massage is to accelerate the healing of the ulcer. Massage is applied mainly around the circumference of the ulcer. The rub and kneading methods are used. At the same time, apply the kneading, pinch, rub-roll, and vibrate methods to the limbs, with a view to improving blood circulation over the whole body.

b) Other treatments: Medical exercise has great value in the prevention and treatment of bedsores. It is also very important to urge the patient to frequently change the position of his body, to keep bedding clean and unwrinkled, and to reduce the pressure on the supporting points of the body as much as possible.

Case History

Li ——, male, age 35, farm-worker. The patient was clinically diagnosed to have myelitis with paraplegia. Because he was confined to bed for a comparatively long period of time, a bedsore was already present on his buttocks. The center of the bedsore had an ulcerated surface two centimeters in diameter. The bottom part of the ulcer and the skin around it were dark and red. The skin lacked elasticity, and had a slight pressure pain. Massage of the skin around the ulcer and of the whole body were given in conjunction with the medical exercise for paraplegia. After about one month or so, the ulcer gradually healed and the patient was recovering from the paraplegia. He asked for discharge from the hospital. Clinical medicinal treatment continued and at the same time the patient's family was told to continue the massage and the medical exercise.

24. Headache

Headache is only a symptom, and can occur in a great number of diseases. However, not all types of headache are suited to the application of massage therapy. For example, headaches resulting from contagious diseases, such as cerebrospinal meningitis, etc. are not suited to this type of treatment. Consequently it is necessary to apply massage therapy selectively in the case of headache.

Etiology

Headache is associated with numerous diseases. In addition to occurring with some contagious diseases and with high fever, headache can occur with common cold, flu, and in certain eye and nose diseases. The patient with high blood pressure often has headache. Moreover, there are also certain chronic, recurring functional headaches, such as migraine and psychosomatic or tension headache.

Symptoms

The headache occurring in common cold and flu is likely to be in the form of an acute attack, with such accompanying symptoms as fever and runny nose.

The headache resulting from eye and nose diseases may be manifested in sub-jective complaints or in objective symptoms of the eye and nose, and com-monly is located in the forehead. Migraine and psychosomatic headache are presented as a chronic process or recur repeatedly, now light and now heavy. Migraine pains occur on one side of the head and are often occompanied by dizziness; psychosomatic or tension headache is felt in both temples, at the back of the head, or at the back of the neck. In the presence of intense headache, both appetite and sleep are affected.

Diagnosis

Headache is only a symptom. In order to make good use of massage therapy a correct diagnosis of the headache's cause is extremely important. First, it is usually necessary to identify acute contagious diseases. Blood pressure must be measured to determine whether hypertension is present. If necessary, a specialist can make an eye and nose examination.

Treatment

Massage therapy is most effective in functional headaches such as migraine, psychosomatic headache, etc. It is also effective in reducing headache symp-toms caused by the common cold and flu. Temporary relief of headache re-sulting from some eye and nose diseases can also be obtained.

a) Massage: (i) The patient usually takes a sitting position. If he cannot sit up, he may take a supine position. The practitioner stands at the patient's head, and the head is wrapped in a towel.

(ii) With the left hand hold the patient's head in place; with the right hand ap-ply a flat-thumb push to the head. First perform a light push massage over the entire head. Then push massage along the mid-line of the head, going from the hairline in front to the hairline at the rear. Do extra pushing at the *baihui* acupoint. First, go from light to heavy, then vice versa. Then the side-of-the-thumb push method can be used to push along both sides of the head, also starting from the front hairline and going to the back hairline. If the patient complains of more discomfort in a certain part of his head, do more pushing there. The above push methods should take about 10 minutes.

(iii) With both thumbs, apply a push massage to the forehead, going from the *yintang* and *zuanzhu* acupoints between the eyebrows to the *taiyang* acupoints in the temples. Or else use the drag method, dragging the thumbs apart from the *yintang* point to the *taiyang* points. At the *taiyang* points, the dig and vibrate methods can be added. After that, drag around the sides of the head to the *fengchi* points behind the ears. For aches in the forehead caused by some eye and nose diseases, even more of these push massages can be applied.

(iv) With the two thumbs, rub and knead both of the *fengchi* acupoints. Then, with the thumb and the first two fingers apply a three-finger pinch going from the back of the head to the nape of the neck. Then use both hands to pinch both *jianjing* acupoints. This process should be repeated several times.

(v) Massage acupoints in the limbs, such as *neiguan*, *hegu*, *zusanli*, and *sanyinjiao*. The finger-dig, finger-vibrate and thumb-tip push methods may be used.

b) Other Treatment: In headaches due to common cold, influenza, eye and nose diseases, or hypertension, after the cause is identified, appropriate medications and other treatments are given.

Therapeutic Effect

After massage the headache patient will feel relaxed and comfortable. After one or several massage-sessions, the headache will subside or disappear.

Case History

Xu ——, male, age 26, technician. He had had paroxysmal headaches for over two years. In the previous month, these had recurred several times. The recurring symptoms were worse than before. The whole head ached, and the pain was especially severe in the back part of the head. When the pain was intense, he experienced a nausea-like sensation, dizziness, and even his sleep was affected. Examination showed blood pressure to be normal and uncovered no specific problems in the eye or nose area. The diagnosis was psychosomatic or tension headache. After one massage using the aforementioned methods, the pain was markedly reduced. After the second massage, the headache completely vanished, and he recovered. A visit to him a short while later found that there had been no recurrence for a month.

Self-massage

(i) Knead the eye-sockets: With the thumb, index, and middle fingers of both hands, knead around both eye sockets in a rotary motion, first turning outward, then inward, 7–8 times each.

(ii) Knead the *taiyang* acupoints: With the tips of the middle fingers of both hands knead both *taiyang* points with a rotary kneading motion, first clockwise, then counter-clockwise, for 7–8 rotations each.

(iii) Drag across the forehead: With the tips of both middle fingers, wipe from between the eyebrows, to the *taiyang* acupoints in the temples, then along both sides of the head to the *fengchi* acupoints at the back hairline.

(iv) Push along the head: With the edge or base of the palms of both hands, firmly press on either side of the head and push from the front hairline to the back hairline. Do this about 30 times.

(v) Pinch the nape of the neck: With the thumb, index, and middle fingers of the right hand pinch from the back of the head downward to the back of the neck. Repeat 5–6 times.

25. Hypertension

This chronic disease normally shows symptoms such as a sensation of enlargement in the head, and dizziness. Measurement of blood pressure shows that it is always maintained above 140 mm of the systolic blood pressure over 90 mm of the diastolic blood pressure on the mercury column. With this disease, a combination of treatments is appropriate in conjunction with massage therapy. A marked therapeutic effect can then be achieved.

Etiology

The causes of this disease are comparatively complex. It can be classified as either secondary or essential hypertension. The former stems from organic diseases, such as of the kidneys, endocrine system or cardiac vessels, and therefore constitutes a specific symptom of these diseases. In essential hypertension, no specific cause can usually be found. This type of hypertension may be related to psychological factors. Of the two types, the most common is primary hypertension. When the disease progresses to its later stages, it can cause structural pathological degeneration (such as of cardiac vessels, brain or kidneys), with serious consequences. The effect of massage therapy is much better where there has been no organic structural degeneration.

Symptoms

In the early stages there may be no subjective symptoms, though generally there are such symptoms as headache, vertigo, a swollen feeling in the head, ringing in the ears, insomnia, flushed face, palpitation and irascibility. In the later stages there may be a sensation of heaviness in the head and lightness in the feet, numbness or swelling of the fingers or toes, tiring easily, poor eyesight, inability to concentrate on work, anorexia, and clear and long urination. In severe cases, the hypertension may bring on paraplegic symptoms caused by cerebral hemorrhage, such as a sudden fall, coma, loss of speech, or partial paralysis.

Diagnosis

Hypertension is diagnosed principally by its symptoms, or by measurement of high blood pressure. The pulse signs are usually wiry, rapid, and leaping. There is a greasy yellow coating on the tongue, and the tongue itself is deep red in color. Sometimes it is necessary to use other methods, such as x-ray, electro-cardiogram, examination of the retina of the eye, and examination of blood chemistry to determine whether or not there is organic structural degeneration.

Treatment

a) Massage: (i) Ask the patient to take a sitting position. Wrap his or her head with a towel. First apply the flat-thumb push to the head. Then push along the forehead and along both sides of the head. The palm press and palm rub methods can also be applied to the head. The whole process requires about 10 minutes. Then apply the finger dig and finger vibrate methods to the *fengchi* acupoints, and the grasp method to the *jianjing* acupoints.

(ii) The flat-thumb push is used on both sides of the back in an up to down direction, covering as wide an area as possible. Then the patient changes to a supine position. With the palm of the hand evenly rub and deeply knead the abdominal area. About 10 minutes is needed to massage both back and abdomen.

(iii) Finally, lightly push and pinch on both lower extremities, combining this with acupoint massage. On the upper limbs, use such points as *hegu*, *shenmen* and *shaohai*, and on the lower limbs, such points as *weizhong*, *chengshan*, *xingjian*, *zusanli*, *sanyinjiao*, *fuliu*, and *yongquan*. In cases where headache and dizziness are important symptoms, apply the finger dig and finger vibrate methods to such points as *xingjian*, *shenmen*, and *shaohai*.

With symptoms such as insomnia, fatigue, anemia, and weakness, make more use of the thumb kneading method on acupoints such as *zusanli*, *sanyinjiao*, *shenmen*, and *yongquan*. In cases with clear and long urination, more pushing on such acupoints as *shenshu* and *mingmen* should be done.

b) *Other Treatment:* In secondary hypertension, treatment should be focused on the underlying cause. In essential hypertension, massage should be combined with medication and physiotherapy to reduce blood pressure. At the same time, a bland diet, regular life and work habits should be followed. Medical exercises for hypertension can also be learned.

Therapeutic Effect

Massage therapy for hypertension can temporarily reduce blood pressure. After the patient has been massaged, his head may feel relaxed and comfortable. In general, there is satisfactory short-term effect, while the long-term effect is uncertain. At the end of the massage treatment, the patient should be taught self-massage and medical exercise that he can keep on with every day. This will contribute to the ultimate consolidation of therapeutic effect.

Case History

Xang ——, female, age 49, cadre. She had a ten-year history of headache, which had in recent years become aggravated, and was accompanied by faintness, insomnia, and sometimes numbness in all four limbs. Blood pressure was measured at 180/100 mm Hg. Examination found no specific pathology in

Self-Massage and Medical Exercise

(i) Push along the head: With the edge or base of the palms of both hands, knead along both sides of the head from the *taiyang* to the *fengchi* acupoints. Then with both thumbs deeply knead *fengchi* until a strong, sore, swelling sensation is felt.

(ii) Knead acupoints: Using left and right thumbs alternately, knead acupoints such as *hegu*, *zusanli*, and *sanyinjiao*, each until it feels sore and swollen. Then chafe the *yongquan* acupoint of each foot, until the sole of the foot becomes warm.

(iii) Knead the abdomen and chafe the lower back: Using left and right palms alternately, do a deep kneading of the abdomen, moving slowly in a clockwise direction. Then, with the hands in fists, press the thumb end of both fists (the "eye" of the fist) against the lower back and chafe up and down until the skin becomes slightly warm.

(iv) Moving the hands: Stand with feet a stride apart and the body's centre of gravity slightly lowered. Raise the hands chest high. First, move the left hand: stretch it out to the left as far as it will go, following it with the eyes and turning the head and trunk as far to the left as possible at the same time. Next, move the right hand: let the hand hang down naturally, the palm turned inward and the fingers slightly bent. With total concentration, and conscious force, pull the right hand slowly across in front of the face and stretch it out to the right. Follow it with the eyes and turn the head and trunk all the way to the right at the same time. Then, move the left hand in the same way as you did the right. Progress slowly in this way, being sure to concentrate and to exert conscious force.

(v) Moving the body: First, take the archer's position, with the left foot forward. Then turn the trunk to the left, raising both arms and bringing the hands together above the head. Follow them with the eyes, bending the head and upper body slightly backward. Then let the arms fall, slowly and naturally, still watching the hands. Switch feet, taking the archer's position with the right foot forward. Perform a similar set of movements to those before, but turning the body to the right instead of the left. In performing these movements, be sure to concentrate fully and to exert conscious force.

the heart or lungs. Blood cholestrol level was rather high. Urine and basal metabolism all measured normal. Hypertension was diagnosed. Drug treatment in combination with massage therapy was adopted. After each massage-session, she reported reduced headache, and lightness and comfort in the head. After 45 massage-sessions, and drug treatment, blood pressure dropped to normal. Her headache, faintness, and insomnia were clearly improved, and she was discharged from hospital.

26. Peptic Ulcer

Ulcer is a common illness of the digestive system. Its cardinal symptom is regular pain in the upper abdominal area. The traditional Chinese doctor calls this "intra-gastric pain."

Etiology

Occurrence of this disease is associated with the effects of psychological factors, overwork, and irregular diet. The pathological changes are chiefly located in the stomach and duodenum.

Symptoms

The disease usually has a chronic course, breaking out from time to time and then clearing up. It is normally most apt to break out in spring and autumn.

(i) Pain in the upper abdomen: At the acute period of an ulcer, except for a few cases without pain, as a rule there is regular pain in the upper abdominal area. Some patients have attacks of pain after eating. Some have attacks when they are hungry, and their pain can usually be relieved by eating. It is most often a burning pain, sometimes referred into the back area. If there is no perforation the pain is generally bearable, though if there is pain at night, it will affect sleep.

(ii) Irregular bowel movements: Most patients have dry movements and only once every 2–3 days. If there is bleeding, then the feces become black. During massive hemorrhage it looks like tar.

(iii) Nausea or vomiting: Vomiting does not generally occur, though if the ulcers are accompanied by pyloric stenosis, vomiting is more apparent, and foods taken in the morning are usually thrown up in the evening.

(iv) Hyperacidity and belching: These symptoms are often seen, especially with peptic ulcers. Ulcers with the complication of pyloric stenosis all present these symptoms, and sometimes the odor of the orally expelled gas is found unpleasant by the patient.

In a small percentage of cases, patients deteriorate to gastric or duodenal bleeding and some ulcers become perforated, leading to acute peritonitis. Late-stage ulcer scar-formation can create pyloric obstruction.

Diagnosis

A preliminary diagnosis can be made based on the history and the typical symptom of pain in the upper abdomen. X-ray examination is helpful in determining the existence and the pathogenic history of the ulcer. Gastric juice analysis can illustrate the condition of gastric secretions: fecal examination can help to show whether the ulcer is bleeding.

With patients who are in extreme pain, it must be determined whether there is perforation or peritonitis. For those with vomiting and belching, it should be determined whether or not pyloric obstruction is present. Moreover, ulcers can sometimes be confused with chronic gastritis or chronic cholecystitis and must be carefully distinguished from them.

Treatment

In adopting massage for treatment of ulcers, therapeutic effect will be better if cases without complications are selected, based on the symptoms and diagnosis outlined above. In cases with perforated ulcer or pyloric obstruction, massage therapy is not suitable. If the patient has massive hemorrhage the practitioner must wait until the bleeding ceases before applying massage.

a) Massage: (i) The patient sits with his hands hanging down and his whole body relaxed or with his hands on the back of a chair and his shoulders turned slightly outward.

(ii) Apply the flat-thumb push along both sides of the vertebral column, going from light to heavy and massaging for about 10 minutes. Hands may be alternated. Then apply the finger dig or bent-finger dig to the pishu and weishu acupoints. Dig until some reaction appears and then switch to the finger vibrate method. End with a light local kneading. Finally the whole back is massaged with the circular-rub method and the palm-heel rub method. The entire procedure takes about 10 minutes.

(iii) The patient then lies face upward, and the therapist massages his abdomen, applying the thumb-dig-method to the *shengwan, zhongwan* and *xiawan* acupoints, being sure to apply just the right amount of force. Do not use this method if there is bleeding and extreme upper-abdominal pain. Follow the rise and fall of breathing: gradually lift the thumb with inhalation, vibrate slowly and dig it in with expiration. Do this about 3–5 times.

If there is gas distension, then apply the single-finger dig and vibrate methods, both using the thumb, to the *tianshu, qihai* and *quonyuan* acupoints.

If bowel movements are irregular, use the palm to do a circular rub of the abdomen, going from the upper right corner around to the lower left corner. The entire abdominal massage should take 3–5 minutes.

(iv) Finally, massage acupoints at some distance from the abdomen. Usually the *hegu* and *zusanli* acupoints on both sides of the body are selected, and the finger-dig and finger vibrate methods are applied until a sore, swollen reaction is produced. If there is severe pain, the *neiguan* and *shenmen* acupoints can also be used. If bowel movements are irregular, acupoints such as *dachangshu* can be used. Skilful adjustments should be made, adding or subtracting acupoints according to symptoms.

b) *Other Treatments:* Other therapeutical measures also should be combined with the massage. Supplementary therapies such as drug therapy, proper rest, avoidance of mental tension, modified diet, and eating less at a time but more frequently are all important. During the period of consolidation after the ulcer has been treated, it is of benefit to teach the patient self-massage and medical exercise, both to be continued over the long term.

Therapeutic Effect

The acute symptoms of a simple ulcer often can soon be relieved or eliminated. After several massage-sessions the desired result can usually be obtained. After healing of the ulcer it is very important to take precautions against its recurrence. During times of year when attacks were previously common, 10–20 massage-sessions can be arranged to prevent the possibility of recurrence. Other measures such as paying attention to diet and persistent practice of self-massage are significant in preventing recurrence.

Case History

Xu ——, male, age 18, high school student. Over a period of a month he had vomited blood three times, so he was hospitalized. For three years the patient had had pain in his upper abdomen and had acid vomitus. He had attacks when he became cold or was under emotional stress. The pain was associated with eating, generally becoming gradually more severe over the 2–3 hours after eating. After he entered the hospital the vomiting of blood ceased. Fecal examination showed a positive occult blood reaction. His face was pale and slightly puffy. Gastric analysis found both ionized acids and total acidity to be somewhat high. An x-ray showed a 0.5 cm concave shadow at the big bend of the stomach. The diagnosis was gastric ulcer.

After he entered the hospital, in addition to regulation of his diet, massage therapy was immediately adopted, as above. After seven days of massage, he reported reduced pain and improved appetite. After a month and a half of treatment, the pain was completely gone. He ate and drank like a normal person and his facial color was back to normal. In order to consolidate the therapeutic effect, massage treatment was continued for a further month and a half, and he was taught self-massage and medical exercise. During this period of time there was no recurrence of the symptoms. X-ray examination showed that the ulcer had completely healed. Body weight had increased by around six kilograms. He was ordered discharged. A month later we made a follow-up visit and found no recurrence.

27. Gastroptosis

This refers to abnormal downward displacement of the stomach. The degree of downward displacement varies greatly. There is often the additional complication of downward displacement of other viscera.

Etiology

A person with a debilitated constitution is prone to having prolapse of the stomach (gastroptosis). Beyond this, an obese person emaciated by a long illness or a woman who has had too many deliveries, are both subject to this condition, because their muscles and other supporting tissues become loose and weak.

Symptoms

The main symptom of gastroptosis is discomfort in the gastric region. Every time the patient eats, there are sensations of swelling, tension, or pressure in the stomach, and often sounds of rumbling water all of which disappear when he or she lies down. There is often belching and a bad taste in the mouth, as well as lack of appetite. The patient seems generally poorly-nourished, depressed, and is easily tired. In the later stages there are also such symptoms as dizziness and insomnia.

Diagnosis

The possibility of this condition should be based on etiology and symptoms, especially when the patient is weak, or tall and thin. It is best to confirm the diagnosis by means of an x-ray and barium-ingestion endoscopic examination.

Treatment

a) *Massage:* (i) First the patient takes a sitting position. Apply the flat-thumb push method along both sides of the spinal column. At the same time, apply the bent-finger dig on the *pishu* and *weishu* acupoints. Then apply the palm-edge chafe method.

(ii) Have the patient take a supine position. The palm-rub method is first applied to the abdominal area. Then with the side of the palm hammer on both sides of the rectus abdominal muscle, hammering just heavily enough to produce contraction reactions in the abdominal muscles. The rate of frequency of the blows should be slow—once every 2–3 seconds. After this knead and rub the lower abdominal area again. If there are such symptoms as abdominal distension, use the index finger to apply the dig message to the *qihai* and *tianshe* acupoints. If appetite is poor, dig at the *zusanli* acupoints.

(iii) Perform the hip-bend method, taking right and left hips alternately. Do it 20–30 times a side, bending the hip with the patient's inhalation and ex-

Medical Exercise

(i) Bend the knees and lift the buttocks: From a supine position, bend the knees and keep the soles of the feet flat on the bed. Raise the buttocks, leaving only the feet and shoulders touching the surface of the bed. (See Diagram 80.) Then tighten the anus and hold that position for about 1 minute. Relax and return to the original position, rest for a moment and repeat, 4–6 times in all.

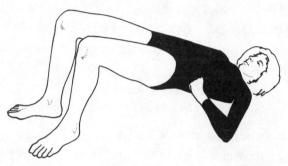

DIAGRAM 80

(ii) Sit up from a supine position: Take a supine position, the lower limbs extended straight and held close together. The upper limbs are grasped behind the head. Using the abdominal muscles, slowly lift the upper part of the body, until a sitting position is reached. Then slowly lie back down again. Rest and repeat, 6–8 times in all.

(iii) Back shoulder-stand: Lie face up, with feet high against a wall and buttocks as close to the wall as possible. The waist should be firmly supported with both hands. Only the shoulders should touch the surface of the bed, and the feet should be flat against the wall. (See Diagram 81.) Maintain this position for about 1 minute, breathing from the abdomen. Rest and repeat, 4 times in all.

tending it with his exhalation. Then do a flat-palm push on the abdomen, sometimes pushing to follow the exhalation, sometimes pushing to cause exhalation.

(iv) If there is dizziness or insomnia, a head-massage should be added in accordance with the symptoms.

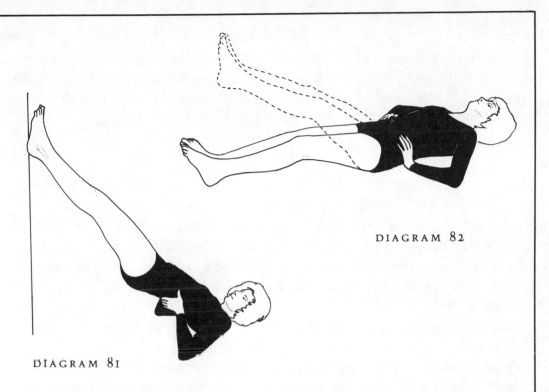

DIAGRAM 82

DIAGRAM 81

(iv) Contract the abdominal muscles and lift both legs: Lie face upward with the legs extended straight and very close together. Using the abdominal muscles, slowly raise both legs together and hold this position for as long as possible. (See Diagram 82.) Lower them slowly, rest, and repeat, 4–6 times in all.

(v) Rub and knead the abdomen with both palms: Lie face upward with both palms on the lower abdomen. Rub and knead the whole abdomen clockwise, going from the lower abdomen upward via the right side of the abdomen, crossing the upper abdomen, and going down the left side of the abdomen to the lower abdomen again. Do this 10–20 times.

b) *Other treatment:* It is best to make use of medical exercise during the application of the massage therapy. Other things, such as paying attention to nutrition, lying down after meals, and avoiding extreme fatigue are also important.

Therapeutic Effect

Massage has an obvious effect on this condition. First, it alleviates the discomfort in the stomach, as well as gradually improving the body's general health. After a period of treatment, various degrees of recovery in the prolapse of the stomach can be seen by x-ray and barium endoscopy.

Case History

Cheng ——, male, age 25, rural cadre. The patient often had pain in the upper abdomen. For five years he had had stomach swelling after meals, and his condition had gradually worsened. During the most recent outbreak, he did not feel like eating at all. Eating only a little was followed by a feeling of fullness, swelling, and pain, and he belched and had bad breath. The patient became quite emaciated. It was finally proved to be gastroptosis by x-ray examination.

As well as applying the massage therapy outlined above, the medical exercise for prolapse of the stomach was used. During the first 2–3 days, he felt that the pain in his upper abdomen had increased, and he also had a feeling of fatigue. Later, he gradually got better, and after two weeks of treatment the pain in the upper abdomen was obviously reduced and his appetite increased. After 48 days of treatment, the pain and other symptoms completely disappeared.

28. Acute Gastroenteritis

Etiology

There can be a number of causes for acute gastroenteritis. What we will deal with here is a kind of acute gastroenteritis that is common in summer and autumn, brought on by carelessness in eating or drinking: eating or drinking too much, drunkenness, eating spoiled food, or food that is too greasy or too spicy, especially when one has a cold. Massage therapy is suitable for treating acute gastroenteritis caused by any of these things. It is not suitable in cases where the acute gastroenteritis has been caused by chemicals (such as strong acids or bases), or is a complication of an infectious disease (such as typhoid fever or dysentery).

Symptoms

The seriousness of the symptoms varies widely. Generally there is nausea, vomiting, swelling of the stomach and a feeling of pressure; and sometimes acute pain, first in the upper abdomen, then in the whole abdominal area, also diarrhea, and anorexia. Moreover, there may be slight fever, dizziness, perspiration, weakening of the limbs, and dry skin. In serious cases there may be dehydration, and the tongue may have a greasy yellow coating. Mild cases last only one or two days but more serious cases may last one or two weeks.

Diagnosis

Diagnosis is relatively easy, and can be made according to history and symptoms. However, if there are symptoms such as fever and pus and blood in the feces, the possibility of dysentery, etc. must be explored, so that treatment of such a condition is not delayed.

Treatment

a) Massage: (i) The patient lies face down, or sits with his or her body bent forward on the table. The area to be massaged must be exposed. An oil or alcohol massage medium can be used.

(ii) Massage is carried out first down the middle and along both sides of the back. First apply the flat-thumb push, then scrape with the side of the thumb. The force used and rate of frequency are gradually increased. Or else use the palm-edge chafe method. In mild cases just massage until the skin is slightly red. In severe cases it is necessary to massage until the skin is more obviously red. The fingers should be frequently dipped into the medium.

(iii) The patient changes to a supine position. Apply the flat-thumb push along the mid-line of the abdomen above the umbilicus and on both sides of the umbilicus until the skin becomes red. The tweak method may also be applied to the abdomen or the back of the neck.

(iv) Finally, on the head area, use the thumbs to apply the divergent push method, starting from the *yintang* or *zuanzhu* acupoint and repeating it about 30–40 times. End by pressing on the *taiyang* point several times.

b) Other Treatment: Concurrently with massage, drug therapy can be used. Bed rest, regulation of diet and keeping warm must also be stressed.

Therapeutic Effect

After one massage-session, the abdominal distention can often be felt to descend, and dizziness is reduced or disappears. At the same time the general symptoms and those in the gastroenteric tract are also improved. This disease generally requires only one massage-session.

Case History

Zhao ——, male, age 40. The patient felt nausea, a desire to vomit and dilation of the stomach. There had been five hours of acute abdominal pain and one diarrhetic bowel movement. Tracing back the history of his disease we found that the disease broke out after he had eaten a great deal of meat and caught cold watching a movie in the open air. Examination showed that his abdomen felt soft and there was a slight pressure pain in the upper abdomen. Slight increase of the peristaltic sound was found by auscultation. The diagnosis was made of acute gastroenteritis. After once applying the above methods of massage, the abdominal swelling was felt to decrease, and the nausea and desire to vomit disappeared. He slept well, was completely recovered the following day, and returned to work.

Folk medicine: Scraping the Back

Use an old copper coin or a porcelain soup spoon. Dip in sesame oil or some other oil and scrape down both sides of the back, from the neck and shoulder area to the waist. Scrape 4–5 strips on either side of the back until the skin becomes red. This method is also called the "cholera-scraping" method.

29. Infantile Indigestion

This is a common infantile disease. Its chief manifestations are disturbed bowel movements and obstructed metabolism. It can be classified according to the seriousness of the symptoms, into simple and toxic indigestion.

Etiology

The digestive organ in the nursing infant is in a state of imperfect development, and its tolerance is comparatively weak. The infant needs relatively more food than an adult does because of its continual growth. Therefore the gastroenteral tract in the infant must put forth a greater effort, and is apt to become exhausted. Aside from this the infant's central nervous system is incompletely developed, and the nerves' regulative functions are not well-established, so maladjustment of metabolism and organic function can easily occur. The causes can be classified into three categories:

a) Improper diet: Feeding too much is one of the most common causes of indigestion. In addition, irregular feeding, insufficient feeding and unsuitable composition of food are all sufficient to cause functional disturbances in the gastroenteral tract, resulting in symtoms such as diarrhea and vomiting.

b) Infection: Infection can in turn be divided into two types: (i) Infection in the digestive tract: Bacteria enter the child's digestive tract with his/her food. This type of infection is most common among bottle-fed infants. E. coli are the most common type of bacteria in such infections.

(ii) Infection outside the digestive tract: In inner ear infections, urinary tract infections, influenza, and respiratory tract infections, bacteria generate toxins that spread through the entire body and cause disturbance of digestive function.

c) Unsuitable climate or environment: Indigestion is most likely to occur during the summer. In hot weather the body excretes too much fluid. If this is not replaced in time, blood circulation is affected, with adverse effects on excretion of wastes. Absorption of toxins produces disturbance of digestive function. The baby is thirsty and sucks too much milk, putting a burden on the digestive tract that it cannot bear. In addition, the adaptive power of the infant is comparatively poor. When the outside temperature is too high, body temperature rises, affecting secretion of gastric acids, and allowing bacteria to breed and multiply easily. At the same time because the body temperature rises and enzymatic activity diminishes, gastroenteral tract function may become abnormal.

Symptoms

a) Simple indigestion: (i) Diarrhea: Bowel movements occur from several times to more than ten times a day. The feces are thin and watery, yellowish-green in colour, with an admixture of some mucus. They have an acid odor and contain small yellowish-green masses. These are saponaceous masses made by chemical combination of salts, such as those of calcium and magnesium, with fatty acids. There is often abdominal swelling.

(ii) Vomiting and regurgitation of milk. Frequency varies.

(iii) Comparative lack of appetite, restlessness and irritability, crying. There is a thin coating on the tongue and weight either does not increase or even decreases.

b) *Toxic indigestion:* Main characteristics are general functional disturbances and the appearance of toxic symptoms.

(i) Frequent vomiting, after drinking water or eating, or even persistent vomiting on an empty stomach.

(ii) Bowel movements increase in number, reaching 15–20 a day. At first the feces contain a large amount of water, mixed with mucus, are yellowish-green, and have an unpleasant odor. Later the bad odor decreases and the fecal masses disappear. The main constituents of the feces become mucus and secretions from the intestinal tract.

(iii) Appetite is poor. The abdomen is obviously swollen. At the same time hyperactivity of the intestinal peristalsis is found. In the late stages, intestinal paralysis occurs.

(iv) The body weight obviously drops, owing to the great amount of water lost. The skin is dry and loses its resilience; the eye sockets are sunken; the anterior fontanelle is low; urine is scanty and yellow. In serious cases the symptoms of acidosis may be present.

(v) Circulatory system: Blood pressure falls; the cardiac sound is not pure; the pulse is rapid and feeble; the skin appears grey; cyanosis can be seen around the lips; the limbs become cold.

(vi) Central nervous system: At first the infant is irritable and restless; then his consciousness becomes clouded; the eyes seldom move; he is indifferent to his surroundings; the hands and feet often present involuntary movements, and convulsions may even appear. When the toxic symptoms continue to develop, the child loses consciousness. He becomes generally debilitated and lapses into a coma.

Diagnosis

Diagnosis is chiefly based on the symptoms and feeding history of the infant. It is also necessary to seek a focus of infection. If possible, the feces should be cultured. It is most important to distinguish this condition from dysentery.

Treatment

a) Massage: The affected infant is held by the mother, or else takes a sitting position. Ginger-juice is prepared for use as a medium.

(i) With the left hand supporting the child's hand, dip the right thumb into the ginger juice. First push along the *pitu* line (See Diagram 83.) Then push upward along the *sanguan* line (See Diagram 84.) Push until the skin becomes red, probably about 200 times or more, alternating hands.

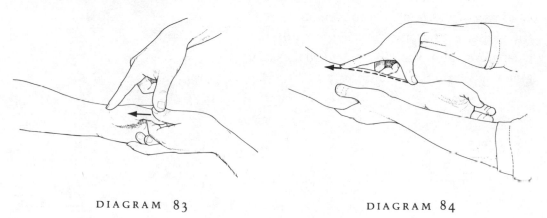

DIAGRAM 83   DIAGRAM 84

(ii) Push down along both sides of the vertebral column, from the seventh cervical vertebra down to the lumbar vertebrae, or apply the spinal pinch method. (See Diagram 79, p. 178.) When the diarrhea is comparatively frequent, add the thumb push method and knead the coccyx. (See Diagram 85.)

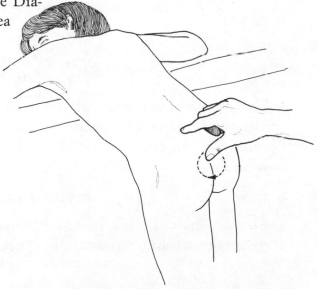

DIAGRAM 85

(iii) With the thumbs apply the divergent push method on both sides of the rib area. Then push on both sides of the umbilicus. If the frequency of watery diarrhea is excessive, knead the umbilicus area with the palm after rubbing the palms together to warm them. Or else apply the grasp method to the *dujiao* points on the abdomen (See Diagram 86).

(iv) Finally apply the finger dig and flat-thumb push methods to the *zusanli* acupoints on both legs.

b) *Other Treatment:* Simultaneously with the massage therapy, proceed with dietary treatment and medication. If necessary, give supplementary liquids.

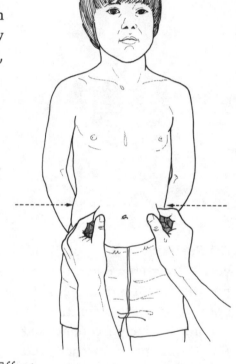

DIAGRAM 86

Therapeutic Effect

Massage is a very good treatment for infantile indigestion. It can gradually alleviate or eliminate the symptoms, and shorten the course of the illness. Results are particularly clear in cases with excessively frequent bowel movements.

Case History

Zhou ——, male, age five months. The patient had run a fever for one day with diarrhea about ten times a day. The diarrhea appeared watery, without pus or blood. He vomited at every feeding. Examination: The abdomen was distended, the eyeballs sunken, the skin dry, and there was medium-grade dehydration. Simple indigestion was diagnosed, and massage therapy was applied as above. On the day following one treatment, bowel movements were reduced to seven. The day after that, there were only four, and abdominal distension was gone. On the third day, diarrhea ceased. Feeding was normal and the patient was discharged.

30. Child Malnutrition

Child malnutrition is a disease involving chronic nutritional imbalance. Its characteristics are insufficient growth of height and weight, and general functional retrogression, especially in higher nerve functions.

Etiology

This condition is usually due to insufficient feeding, and is most often seen among bottle-fed babies. It can also be the result of improper feeding, usually of a premature baby. The disease manifests itself as well in infants with chronic indigestion, and those who consume too much during a long-term illness. In addition to these, the disease can be caused by congenital deformities such as harelip and cleft palate which make feeding difficult; by constitutional abnormalities; also by poor environment, such as lack of sunlight or exercise.

Symptoms

The main features of this disease are: the infant becomes thin; body weight either does not increase or even decreases; subcutaneous fat diminishes or disappears. Clinically it can be classified into three degrees according to the seriousness of the symptoms:

First-degree malnutrition: Fat is still stored in every part of the body, but the subcutaneous fat layers of the abdomen and of the trunk become thin. Muscle growth is very poor. Skin color is normal or pale. Body weight is 10–20% less than normal, but height remains unchanged. Body temperature is normal and general condition remains good.

Second-degree malnutrition: Body weight is 20–30% less than normal and height is 1–3 cm less than normal. The subcutaneous layers of fat in the trunk, limbs, and hips, disappear; the skin loses its resilience and becomes pale, loose, dry, and wrinkled; hair grows thin and dry; the face becomes thin; muscle tone is reduced or increased. Motor functions develop slowly and the infant cannot stand or walk.

Third-degree malnutrition: The body weight is 40 or 50% less than normal and height is also lower than normal. The skin is dry, appears grey or sometimes bluish-purple, loses its resilience, and forms thin, wrinkled folds. Fat disappears from the face; the eyes become sunken; the forehead is marked with wrinkles. The cheeks become hollow and the cheekbone protrudes; the chin becomes pointed. The child looks like a little old man or old woman. Innumerable wrinkles form on the skin of the trunk and limbs; the flesh becomes thin, the abdomen becomes sunken or bloated. In serious cases, the child becomes dehydrated, and the fontanelle sinks inward.

The infant with second or third degree dystrophy may have anorexia. His or her tolerance of foods may be low, and there may be constipation or diarrhea. The child may be irritable and cry easily, he or she may show little energy, and may be restless during sleep. Cardiac sound may be dull; the rhythm of the heart slow; body temperature lower than normal; a variety of vitamin-deficiency symptoms may appear. Because resistance is low, he or she will be susceptible to such disorders as upper respiratory tract infection, influenza, bronchitis, pneumonia, inner ear infections, dermatitis, and urinary tract infections.

Diagnosis

Diagnosis can be made based upon the symptoms mentioned above. But in each case the cause of the pathology must be sought, and chronic infections such as tuberculosis, chronic dysentery, and parasitic diseases must be excluded.

Treatment

a) Massage: (i) Have the affected child held by its mother. After dipping them in ginger juice, use the thumbs to push along the *pitu* and *sanguan* lines of both arms, returning along the *liufu* line. Push 100–200 times along each line. Then knead and push with the thumbs on the *zusanli* acupoints of both legs.

(ii) Massage other points according to each patient's various symptoms. If there is abdominal swelling, constipation or loose bowels, push along both sides of the umbilical area and knead the umbilicus and the coccyx. If there is slight fever, apply a push massage at the *dahengwen* points on the hands, knead the *neilaogong* in the palms and push at the *tianheshui* point of the elbow. If there are chills, cough and fever, then push at the *feishu* point and along both sides of the spinal column, and apply a dig massage at *ershanmen*, *errenshangma*, and *yiwofeng* on the hands.

b) Other Treatment: In addition to massage therapy, it is important to eliminate the causes of the disease. Regulation of nutrition and improvement of the method of feeding are both important. In addition, more exposure to sunlight, and medical exercise, can both be used.

Therapeutic Effect

Massage can usually rapidly improve the appetite of the affected child and increase resistance to disease, bringing about a gradual return to health.

Case History

Ma ——, one year old boy. Because of a lack of milk and improper feeding, the patient had often been ill since birth. He was thin and cried often. Over the previous two weeks, his illness had become more serious. His crying became weaker, his eyes were seldom open, and his limbs were puffy. As a result, he was admitted to hospital. Examination: Growth and nutrition were both very poor. He was small and weak and showed little energy. His anterior fontanelle was not yet closed. His face was yellowish and slightly pasty, cheeks reddish and lips dark red. His tongue lacked moisture, had a slight yellow coating and was dry. There was ulceration at the corner of the left eye. The abdominal area was swollen and the lower limbs slightly puffy. A diagnosis of malnutrition was made.

After blood transfusion, medication and dietary treatment, his condition was somewhat improved. Massage as above was begun on his 12th day in hospital. After 25 treatments, the general situation was good. Appetite was obviously increased. Body temperature was steady. Excretion and urination were normal. He showed more energy. The face and the whole body were plumper than they had been before treatment. Body weight had increased.

There was neither puffiness nor dehydration. He had basically completely re-covered, so treatment was stopped.

31. Child Pneumonia

Child pneumonia is a general term for inflammatory pathological changes in the lungs. According to clinical features and features of pathological anatomy it is divided into primary and secondary pneumonia, and bronchial and lobar pneumonia. The massage used varies little from type to type, so we will illus-trate with the most frequently seen type, which is bronchial pneumonia.

Etiology

This disease is caused by pathogens (such as bacteria and viruses) attacking the lungs. The child's health and nutritional condition are also significant. Children debilitated by a long illness are more susceptible to the disease, and their symptoms and pathological changes are more serious. Therefore the tra-ditional Chinese doctor considers that the disease is caused by internal injury and external susceptibility. Clinically, the traditional doctor distinguishes cases as involving deficiency or fullness, and cold or heat.

Symptoms

Generally there is a sudden high fever up to around 40°C, accompanied by cough, rapid breathing, etc. The cough is usually intense, sometimes with vomiting. The symptom of rapid breathing sets in suddenly, and generally there is agitation of the jaw muscles. At the same time there can be such phenomena as facial pallor and bluish-purple lips. In addition, because of dif-ferences in the severity of symptoms, there can be somnolence, restlessness, irritability or even unconsciousness. In serious cases there are convulsions and coma.

Diagnosis

There is no difficulty in making a diagnosis by etiology and symptoms. Aus-cultation of the lungs will show dry and wet rales, and sometimes there will be inspiratory sounds in the bronchus. An x-ray will show flat, dark points of shadow of various sizes. All these can help confirm the diagnosis and dis-criminate specific conditions. Examining the patterns of the skin on the child's fingers can also be helpful in selecting specific treatments to apply. The patterns are usually purple or bluish-purple and this colour goes beyond the *qiguan* or *mingguan* point. If the patterns are blue and the colour goes beyond the *mingguan* point, prognosis is usually poor.

Treatment

No matter what type of pneumonia it may be, and no matter whether it is acute or deferred pneumonia, massage may be applied as an accessory treatment.

a) Massage: General method and sequence: (i) Have the affected child held by someone or place it in a lying position. Prepare some medium such as raw ginger juice. First push along the *pitu* and *sanguan* lines. Then apply a divergent push on both the palms and the dorsal sides of both hands and knead the *wailaogong* point.

(ii) Expose the chest and back. First apply a push massage at the *fengchi, fengfu, duzhui* and *feishu* points on the back. Then push at the *rupang, rugen,* and *shanzhong* points.

(iii) Then massage distant acupoints, for instance pushing and kneading at the *jiexi, yongquan,* and *zusanli* acupoints of the lower legs and feet.

(iv) End the massage by pushing at the *yintang, taiyin,* and *taiyang* points. The complete course of massage should take 20 minutes or so.

Methods for specific situations:

(i) If there is high fever, push at the *tianheshui* point as well.

(ii) If there is fever but no perspiration push again along the *sanguan* line and apply a grasp massage at both *jianging* and *neilaogong.*

(iii) If there is rapid breathing, agitation and hypoxia, then push at the *fengchi, fengfu, fengmen, dazhui, feishu* and *rangu* acupoints, then at the other sites.

(iv) If a great deal of rale is discovered by auscultation of the lungs, and if the patient has a strong constitution and has only been ill for a short time, then pushing may be concentrated at *feishu* and *sanguan.* If the patient has a weak constitution and has been ill for a longer period of time, and if it is secondary pneumonia, then do more pushing along *pitu* and on the back.

(v) When there are digestive-tract symptoms, such as diarrhea, rub the abdomen and apply a push massage at the coccyx. When there is vomiting, push *banmen* as well.

b) Other Treatment: In treatment of child pneumonia massage is only one of the accessory therapies in a combined treatment. Clinically, the use of antibiotics is still most important. At the same time, other kinds of treatment should also be used.

Therapeutic Effect

If massage is used as part of the comprehensive treatment of this illness, therapeutic effect is often more satisfactory and the course of the illness is shortened. Especially in deferred pneumonia, massage can often cause rales and other symptoms to disappear sooner.

Case History

Zhang ——, one year old female. The patient was hospitalized because she had suffered from high fever for two days and rapid breathing for one day. She was agitated with bluish facial color and had labored breathing. By auscultation the lungs were found to be full of dry and wet rales. The skin-patterns of the fingers were blue, even beyond the *qiguan* point. A clinical diagnosis of bronchial pneumonia was made. In addition to antibiotics and oxygen treatment, massage therapy was given. After two treatments the rapid breathing was calmed, and the rales in the lungs were reduced. After eight treatments the rales completely disappeared. Body weight and appetite returned to normal and she was discharged.

Folk Medicine: Rubbing the back with raw ginger

Have the back area of the affected child exposed. Take a piece of raw ginger. Peel one end of the ginger and pare it to a smooth, round surface. Dip the peeled end of the ginger into warm water and rub up and down both sides of the child's back, generally starting from the lower cervical vertebrae and going down to the lumbar area. Rub most at the *dazhui* point and at the *sho* points of the upper back (such as *feishu*, *xinshu*, *geshu*). Rub until the skin becomes slightly red.

APPENDIX 1

SELF-MASSAGE FOR STRENGTHENING THE BODY AND PREVENTING DISEASE

1. Knock on the teeth: With the lips gently closed, use the tips of the fingers to knock rhythmically against the lower and the upper teeth 30–40 times each.

2. Clean the mouth: With the lips gently closed, use the tongue to forcefully wipe out around the space between the teeth and the lips. Wipe around to the left and to the right 30 times each.

3. Rub the hands: Rub the palms together 30–40 times, with increasing speed, until they become warm.

4. Rub the face: Rub the face with the warmed palms, first going from the left side of the face across the forehead to the right side 7–8 times.

5. Knead the eyes: With the knuckles of the index, middle, and ring fingers of both hands, knead with a circular motion around the eyesockets, first going from the inside corner to the outside, then from the outside corner to the inside, 7–8 times each.

6. Knead *taiyang*: With the tips of the middle fingers of the left and right hands, press on the *taiyang* acupoints in the left and right temples and knead with a circular motion, first clockwise and then counter-clockwise, 7–8 times each.

7. Wipe the forehead: With the tips of the middle finger of both hands, wipe from between the eyebrows out toward both sides, gradually reaching the hairline.

8. Push on the head: With the sides or bases of the palms of both hands, press against the sides of the head, then push from the front hairline to the back hairline. Do this 30–40 times.

9. Dig at *baihui*, *fengfu*, and *dazhui:* Dig and then knead at each of these three acupoints, spending about 1 minute at each.

10. Vibrate the ears: With the fingers of both hands against the back of the head, cover the ear canals with the palms and make a quick, rhythmic drumming notion, about 30–40 times.

11. Knock behind the ears: With the fingers of both hands against the back of the head, and the palms tightly covering the ear canals, tap against the back of the head with the index and middle fingers, so that a "dong" sound is heard. Do this about 20 times.

12. Pat the chest: Spread the fingers of both hands and tap against the chest with the flats of the fingers, inhaling with each tap. Do this about 7–8 times.

13. Chafe the ribs: Use the outside edges of the hands to chafe the two sides of the rib-cage quickly 30–40 times.

14. Knead the abdomen: Press on the umbilical area with the left hand and press down on the back of the left hand with the right. Then deeply and forcefully knead the abdomen, going clockwise 30–80 times.

15. Chafe the lumbar area: With the hands in fists, use the thumb-end of the fists (the "eye" of the fist) to chafe up and down quickly and forcefully on both sides of the lumbar region about 30–40 times.

16. Hammer the spine and the sacrum: With the hands in fists, hammer along both sides of the spine, starting from as high you can reach and going down as far as the coccyx. Do this 3–4 times.

17. Rub-roll the thighs: Sit with legs folded and rub-roll each thigh with the palms of both hands, 30–40 times.

18. Pinch the calves: Sitting with legs folded apply a pinch massage to the gastrocnemius muscle of the back of the calf, going from the top of the muscle down to the Achilles tendon. Do the left leg first, then the right.

19. Chafe *yongquan:* Quickly and forcefully chafe the *yongquan* acupoints of the sole of the foot with the outside edge of the hand. Chafe 30–40 times, until the center of the foot is warm. Do the left foot first.

20. Breathing exercise: Stand with the legs shoulder-width apart. Lift the hands from the abdominal region upward to the throat, simultaneously lifting the head, bending backward at the waist and breathing in. Then draw the hands downward from the throat back to the abdomen, lower the head, bend forward at the waist and breathe out. As you breathe out, make the sounds "ha-ho-hee-hoo." Repeat the exercise twice.

Self-massage is not only used to strengthen the body and prevent disease, but it can also be useful in actually treating disease and in consolidating the effect of other therapies. The 20 massage methods outlined above can be used as a group or certain of them can be selected, according to specific circumstances. When used preventatively, they can be done in the morning after rising, or at night just before going to bed. When used during recuperation from illness, certain of them can be selected, according to one's condition. In disease that affects the senses, massage of the head area may be emphasized. In those that affect the lower limbs, massage of the legs is even more important. And so on.

APPENDIX 2

EYE-CARE MASSAGE

1. Knead the upper corners of the eyesockets: With the flats of the thumbs, press against the upper inside corners of the eyesockets, below the eyebrows (at the *tianying* point). The fingers should be slightly bent and propped against the forehead. Gently knead at the *tianying point*.

2. Squeeze and press the base of the nose: With the thumb and index finger of one hand, squeeze the base of the nose (at the *jingming* acupoint). First press down, then squeeze upward, alternating these motions.

3. Knead the cheeks: With the flats of the index fingers, press on the center of each cheek (at about the *sibai* acupoint). Hook the thumbs into the depression under the lower jaw and clench the rest of the fingers. Knead the centers of the cheeks with the index fingers.

4. Scrape the eyesockets: Slightly bend the index fingers and press the side of the second knuckle against the top of the eyesocket. Press the thumbs against the *taiyang* acupoints in the temples and clench the other three fingers. Scrape downward around the eyesockets with the index fingers while kneading hard on the *taiyang* points with the thumbs.

These massages should be done 20 times each, both in the morning and at night. They can also be done after looking at something for a long time, for instance after prolonged reading.

APPENDIX 3

MASSAGE METHODS

1. **Press Method** . . . . ànfǎ
   palm press method . . . . zhǎng ànfǎ
   finger press method . . . . zhǐ ànfǎ
   two-palm opposed press method . . . . shuāngzhǎng duìànfǎ
   two-thumb opposed press method . . . . shuāngzhǐ duìànfǎ
   elbow press method . . . . zhǒu ànfǎ
2. **Rub Method** . . . . mófǎ
   thumb rub method . . . . zhǐ mófǎ
   two-thumb rub method . . . . shuāngshoǔ zhǐ mófǎ
   two-thumb circular rub method . . . . shuāngshoǔ mǔzhǐ
                                                                                   huímófǎ
   palm rub method . . . . zhǎng mófǎ
   palm-heel rub method . . . . zhǎnggēn mófǎ
3. **Push Method** . . . . tuīfǎ
   flat-thumb push method . . . . mǔzhǐpíng tuīfǎ
   spiral push method . . . . luówén tuīfǎ
   divergent push method . . . . fēntuīfǎ
   side-of-the-thumb push method . . . . mǔzhǐcè tuīfǎ
   shaoshang push method . . . . shàoshāng tuīfǎ
   thumb-tip push method . . . . mǔzhǐjiān tuīfǎ
   flat-palm push method . . . . zhǎngpíng tuīfǎ
   palm-heel push method . . . . zhǎnggēn tuīfǎ

4. **Grasp Method** . . . . náfǎ
   three-finger grasp method . . . . sānzhǐ náfǎ
   five-finger grasp method . . . . wǔzhǐ náfǎ
   shaking grasp method . . . . dǒudòng náfǎ
   muscle-snapping method . . . . tánjīn fǎ
5. **Roll Method** . . . . gǔnfǎ
   roller roll method . . . . gǔnzhóu gǔnfǎ
6. **Dig Method** . . . . qiāfǎ
   single-finger dig method . . . . dānzhǐ qiāfǎ
   bent-finger dig method . . . . qūzhǐ qiāfa
   finger-cut method . . . . zhǐqiē fǎ
7. **Pluck Method** . . . . bōfǎ
   energy-system pluck method . . . . bōluò fǎ
8. **Kneading Method** . . . . róufǎ
   thumb kneading method . . . . zhǐ róufǎ
   palm kneading method . . . . zhǎng róufǎ
   palm-heel kneading method . . . . zhǎnggēn róufǎ
9. **Vibrate Method** . . . . zhènfǎ
   finger vibrate method . . . . zhǐ zhènfǎ
   palm vibrate method . . . . zhǎng zhènfǎ
   electric vibrate method . . . . diànzhènfǎ
10. **Drag Method** . . . . māfǎ
    muscle-straightening method . . . . lǐjīn fa
11. **Chafe Method** . . . . cāfǎ
    finger chafe method . . . . zhǐ cāfa
    palm-edge chafe method . . . . zhǎngcè cāfǎ
12. **Rub-roll Method** . . . . cuōfǎ
    palm rub-roll method . . . . zhǎng cuōfa
    palm-edge rub-roll method . . . . zhangcè cuōfǎ
13. **Pinch Method** . . . . niēfǎ
    three-finger pinch method . . . . sānzhǐ niēfǎ
    five-finger pinch method . . . . wuzhǐ niēfǎ
    spinal pinch method . . . . niējí fǎ
14. **Tweak Method** . . . . chěfǎ
    twist method . . . . nìngfǎ

15. **Flick Method** . . . . tánfǎ
16. **Knock Method** . . . . kòufǎ
    middle-finger knock method . . . . zhōngzhǐ kòufǎ
    five-finger knock method . . . . wǔzhǐ kòufǎ
17. **Pat Method** . . . . páifǎ
    finger pat method . . . . zhǐ páifǎ
    back-of-the-fingers pat method . . . . zhǐbèi páifǎ
    palm pat method . . . . zhǎng páifǎ
18. **Hammer Method** . . . . chuífǎ
    prone-fist hammer method . . . . wòquán chuífǎ
    upright-fist hammer method . . . . zhíquán chuífǎ
    palm-edge hammer method . . . . zhǎngcè chuífǎ
19. **Extension Method** . . . . shēnfǎ
    shoulder extension method . . . . shēnjiān fǎ
    elbow extension method . . . . shēnzhǒu fǎ
20. **Bend Method** . . . . qufǎ
    calf bend method . . . . qūxiǎotuǐ fǎ
    hip bend method . . . . qūkuān fǎ
    two-hip bend method . . . . shuāngqukuān fǎ
21. **Rotation Method** . . . . yáofǎ
    neck rotation method . . . . yáojǐng fǎ
    shoulder rotation method . . . . yáojiān fǎ
    hip rotation method . . . . yáokuān fǎ
    lumbar rotation method . . . . yáoyāo fǎ
22. **Shake Method** . . . . dǒufǎ
    upper-limb shake method . . . . dǒushàngzhī fǎ
    lower-limb shake method . . . . dǒuxiàzhī fǎ
23. **Stretch Method** . . . . yǐnshēnfǎ
    lumbar stretch method . . . . yāo yǐnshēnfǎ
    upper-limb stretch method . . . . shàngzhī yǐnshēnfǎ
    lower-limb stretch method . . . . xiàzhī yǐnshēnfǎ
    moving the leg . . . . bāntuǐ
24. **Treading Method** . . . . cǎifǎ

APPENDIX 4

TABLE OF WEIGHTS AND MEASURES

Weight:

1 catty (*jin*) = 10 *liang* = 500 grams = 1.1 pounds

1 *liang* = 10 *fen* = 50 grams = 1¾ ounces

1 *qian* = ⅒ liang

Distance:

1 *li* = ½ kilometer = ⅓ mile

Approximate liquid measure:

2 catties of water = 1 liter = 1.1 quarts = 1 kilogram

APPENDIX 5

TABLE OF ACUPOINTS

I = Heart meridian; II = Small intestine meridian; III = Bladder meridian; IV = Kidney meridian; V = Pericardium meridian; VI = Three heater meridian; VII = Gall bladder meridian; VIII = Liver meridian; IX = Lung meridian; X = Large intestine meridian; XI = Stomach meridian; XII = Spleen meridian.

Chinese Name	Translation of Chinese Name	Numerical Point
Baihui	hundred meetings	Governor Vessel 20
Yintang	hall of the imprint	an extra point
Taiyang	highest *yang*	an extra point
Jingming	eyes bright	III-1
Zuanzhu	collecting bamboo	III-2
Sibai	four-white	XI-2
Tinggong	listening palace	II-19
Tinghui	hearing meeting	VII-2
Yifeng	screens the wind	VI-17
Yingxiang	welcomes fragrance	X-20
Renzhong	person-middle	Governor Vessel 26
Jianyu	shoulder *yu* point	X-15
Chize	foot marsh	IX-5
Quchi	crooked pond	X-11
Shaohai	little sea	I-3
Shousanli	hand three miles	X-10

Neiguan	inner pass	v-6
Waiguan	outer pass	VI-5
Lieque	narrow defile	IX-7
Hegu	joining of the valleys	X-4
Yangxi	*yang* stream	X-5
Yangchi	*yang* pond	VI-4
Yanggu	*yang* valley	II-5
Shenmen	spirit gate	I-7
Daling	great mound	v-7
Taiyuan	great abyss	IX-9
Ten xuan	ten *xuan* points	
Quepen	broken basin	XI-12
Zhongfu	middle palace	IX-1
Rugen	breast root	XI-18
Shangwan	upper stomach cavity	CV (Conception Vessel) 13
Zhongwan	middle stomach cavity	CV-12
Xiawan	lower stomach cavity	CV-10
Shenque	spirit deficiency	CV-8
Qihai	sea of *qi* (energy)	CV-6
Guanyan	origin of the passes	CVU-4
Tianshu	heavenly pivot	XI-25
Qichong	*qi* rushing	XI-30
Fengchi	wind pond	VII-20
Fengfu	wind palace	GV (governor vessel) 16
Yamen	gate of dumbness	GV-15
Dazhui	great hammer	GV-14
Fengmen	wind gate	III-12
Feishu	lungs correspondence	III-13
Xinshu	heart correspondence	III-15
Geshu	diaphragm correspondence	III-17
Ganshu	liver correspondence	III-18
Danshu	gall bladder correspondence	III-19
Pishu	spleen correspondence	III-20
Weishu	stomach correspondence	III-21
Shenshu	kidney correspondence	III-23

Dachangshu	large intestine correspondence	III-25
Shangliao	upper *liao* point	III-31
Ciliao	second *liao* point	III-32
Zhongliao	middle *liao* point	
Xialiao	lower *liao* point	
Mingmen	gate of life	GV-4
Yangguan	*yang* pass	GV-3
Jianjing	shoulder well	VII-21
Jianliao	shoulder *liao* point	VI-15
Jianzhen	upright shoulder	II-9
Tianzong	heavenly ancestor	II-11
Gaohuang	richness for the vitals	III-38
Huantiao	jumping circle	VII-30
Chengfu	support and hold up	III-50
Xuehai	sea of blood	XII-10
Xiyan	knee-eye	
Zusanli	foot three miles	XI-36
Yanglingquan	*yang* mound spring	VII-34
Juegu	bone separation	VII-39
Kunlun	*kunlun* mountains	III-60
Pucan	servants aide	III-61
Yinlingquan	*yin* mound spring	XII-9
Sanyinjiao	three *yin* crossing	XII-6
Jiexi	released stream	XI-41
Taixi	great stream	IV-3
Taichong	supreme rushing	VIII-3
Chongyang	rushing *yang*	XI-42
Weizhong	accepting middle	III-54
Chengjin	supporting muscle	
Chengshan	supporting mountain	III-57
Yongquan	bubbling spring	IV-1

INDEX